The Childhood Trauma Recovery Workbook for Adults

Interactive Exercises, Therapeutic Prompts, and CBT/DBT Strategies for Dealing with Depression, Anxiety, Shame, and Other Effects of Abuse

Norman J. Fried, PhD, and Nathan Spiteri

ULYSSES PRESS

Published by:
Ulysses Press
PO Box 3440
Berkeley, CA 94703
www.ulyssespress.com

ISBN: 978-1-64604-625-6

Printed in the United States
10 9 8 7 6 5 4 3 2 1

Acquisitions editor: Shelona Belfon
Managing editor: Claire Chun
Editor: Renee Rutledge
Proofreader: Barbara Schultz
Front cover design: Ashley Prine
Interior design and layout: Jake Flaherty Design
Artwork: leaf pattern © Apostrophe/shutterstock.com

Contents

Introduction

As we grow through childhood, we hope to gain a sense of mastery over the world around us. Many of us live under the illusion that the future is ours for the taking, and that any hardships we confront along the way will work out well in the end. But some of us were raised in homes where emotional harm and/or physical abuse prevailed. We were hurt emotionally, physically, and even sexually. As a result, we developed a belief that the world is a dangerous place. We learned to surrender to the words and actions of caretakers or authority figures who made us see life through their negative, even hateful, eyes. Fear and trauma ignited deep within us, and we developed maladaptive ways of coping. As a result, the promise of a future filled with safety, security, and infinite opportunities for success turned into a myth or dream that only happened in other children's lives.

Our attempts at healing are varied but often not successfully achieved. This is because healing from child abuse defies most typical efforts at psychotherapy, for the path to healthy functioning requires the expert understanding of a professional fluent in the language of trauma and loss. As survivors of abuse, we experience difficulties with our sense of self. We waver in our ability to trust in others, and we often find ourselves in relationships that are challenged by a fear of abandonment. This is happening because, at an age when our basic human needs for safety and security were supposed to be met, some of us experienced a rupture in the moral codes that were meant to keep us safe. Devoid of physical, emotional, and even sexual boundaries, we had little recourse but to submerge into an inner world of fear, confusion, and self-blame. Doubt, anger, guilt, and shame all began to coalesce beneath the surface of our seemingly normal childhood; but we felt far from normal on the inside.

These complicated emotions were eventually directed toward family members who accidentally activated, or "triggered," our fear of closeness. To escape these emotions, some of us learned to become numb. We were seemingly able to "switch off" the noise around us and make our inner world fall to silence. Or, we may have felt as if we were breaking into small pieces. Fragmented memories and unexpected flashbacks developed, creating a sense that we were out of control. In the aggregate, all of us who were hurt as children experienced a loss of direction. Robbed of a safe home base, the future took on a new and uncharted course.

If this describes some of your experiences or emotions growing up, then this workbook is for you. Guided by cognitive behavioral theory, as well as narrative (post-modern) approaches to psychotherapy, this guide is designed to help you examine your own life stories and attempt to imbue them with new meaning. The goal is for you to become the expert of your own story. You will be given the chance to honor your own thoughts, feelings, and actions from new and healthier perspectives, so you may begin to recover your sense of identity and authenticity.

How to Use This Workbook

The curriculum in this workbook is written in an easy-to-use, personal format that is designed to educate and guide you as you embark on your healing journey. Each of the ten chapters contains important clinical information about child abuse, its effect on us as growing humans, and ways that we can all rise above our pain and sorrow. Embedded within the clinical content are thought-provoking questions that you will be prompted to answer, as well as mindfulness exercises that you can employ, as you move through the process. Take the time you need to respond to the questions and the exercises, and to reflect on how these activities make you feel. The process is to be approached at whatever pace feels right to you. Awareness comes slowly, and it requires patience and loving-kindness.

We (the authors) recommend that you go through the chapters in order, giving yourself time to process and reflect on the emotions that may arise. You may find it helpful to repeat some of the exercises or answer the questions several times. You may even discover that you want to spend extra time on a particular topic. This is your program. Take the time you need and remember, no one else has to read or listen to your personal work here unless you wish to share it. The journey upon which you are embarking respects that you are always the one in control.

Recovery from the trauma of child abuse is a delicate and loving process between patient and counselor, and the healing travels in both directions. You, the reader, have a story to tell—a story that is not only filled with pain, but also with wisdom and healing potential. We, the writers, have our own stories to tell, for we too are survivors. We will be with you as you work through the emotional material that lies before you. In working together like coauthors, a new story is being born, a story of self-love and love for others.

If you discover that you are feeling **triggered,** or emotionally activated, by any of the material, please remember to take a break. The information provided in this workbook can be highly stimulating. Thus, watch your pace; close the book when necessary and return when you feel strong again. In this manner, you will discover the therapeutic value that is inherent in the work.

It is also a good idea, if you are feeling triggered, to reach out to a trusted friend, counselor, psychologist, or psychiatrist. When we allow our story to be heard by someone who has the ability to understand our pain, we discover the healing power of community. Do not be afraid to ask for help.

The theories, questions, and mindfulness techniques we offer in this workbook reflect our learnings from over 30 years of trauma therapy practice. In addition to the academic and empirical data offered, we provide wisdom gained through lived experience. Many lessons were learned through the hardships of surviving our own traumas, and from doing the work to heal. In addition, our patients and colleagues, as well as the pioneering work of esteemed leaders in the field of trauma research and therapy, have been our teachers. Specifically, interested readers are referred to the illustrious work of Erich Fromm, MD; Beverly James, LCSW; Judith Lewis Herman, MD; Bessel van der Kolk, MD; Marsha Linehan, MD; and journalist and writer Terry Philpot. In addition, we reference the spiritual and philosophical theories of Martin Buber, Viktor Frankl, and Carl Jung.

Tips for Practice

As you work your way through this book, keep several helpful points in mind:

- Consider creating a schedule of when you will read and work through a chapter. This suggestion comes from research on **emotion regulation**, or the ability to control our emotional state. Specifically, when we are faced with a seemingly unending set of stimuli, we are more prone to feel anxious and out of control. The more we organize our day, the better we feel. Therefore, create a structured plan for approaching this work. You will be more capable of regulating the feelings of anxiety that may arise.

- You will be introduced to many new exercises and techniques for addressing your deep feelings from the past. Allow ample time to digest the content of each question and exercise. Remember, the questions and exercises are guidelines only. Feel free to adapt them in ways that work best for you.

- After completing an exercise, consider closing the book and reflecting upon what you just experienced. Offer yourself moments of self-care, which may include a long walk or other ways of experiencing the elements of nature. Research reveals that this helps to oxygenate the blood and rejuvenate the neurotransmitters in the brain.[1]

- Take your time. This is not a course of study that comes with a final examination, nor is there a graduation day. Every day offers new opportunities for learning and growing. If you push yourself too hard or read through the material too quickly, it will likely not offer you the benefits you seek.

- You may feel a need to pass over sections of the material that provoke discomfort. This is okay. You can always come back to them later if you wish.

- You may want to do some of these exercises, or answer some of the questions, in the presence of a therapist. This may allow you the opportunity to dig deeper into a memory or feeling, and you will have the support and guidance of a trained professional to help structure your exploration.

- If you do not attend psychotherapy, consider reaching out to a therapist for a few sessions. Developing a therapeutic alliance reminds us that we are not alone on this journey, and it ensures that the path we are on will contain the wisdom of someone who knows the way.

- We encourage you to read additional material relating to the issues that arise through your healing journey. This increases your awareness and allows you to develop greater skills acquisition.

- There is no wrong way to answer the questions in this book. The journey you are undertaking is an initiation into a new way of living. You are reading this book because you are interested in gaining the wisdom that comes through facing pain. And this is a courageous decision. If you think you are doing any of the work wrong, just remember: It is a *downward* path toward growing *up*.[2] The way to healing is not always the typical; but as long as you stay the path, you are healing.

- Maintain contact with people who have been through a similar journey. Establishing healthy and nurturing relationships breaks the constriction and isolation you may feel when you are working through past traumas. Support groups have been established and designed for survivors of child abuse. Some are quite helpful for they offer a chance to speak a common language with others who are, or once were, in a similar place.

- Do not be surprised if you run into resistance from friends who do not understand this journey. Many will tell you to "get over" the pain, rather than appreciate your need to "get through it." Try to find solace in the presence of one friend who understands your involuntary, almost compulsive, need to journey through the darkness to a place of light.
- In telling your story in a safe context, you will discover the love that comes from honest sharing. Try to gift your healthy friends with your love and allow them to honor you with their love in return. You are growing and learning, changing into a healthier version of yourself. The work is hard, but the rewards are many, for the love that awaits you is filled with the light you were always meant to receive.

As You Begin Your Journey

The development of the material in this workbook is the result of our continued efforts to grow through our own journeys of recovery. It is our willingness to share our experiences, as well as the wisdom we have gained along the way, that has made this project a reality. Our belief is that healing is possible. When we commit to the work, connect with others who were once where we are now, and hold onto a faith in a higher power or a higher self, we will discover the transformation that healthy love creates.

1

Anger and Hatred

If you are patient in one moment of anger, you will escape a hundred days of sorrow.

Chinese Proverb

Anger and hatred are two emotions that every one of us lives with throughout our entire lives, particularly those of us who have experienced a trauma at a young age. The inner world of the healthy child starts with wonder and faith in the goodness of a safe world. But many of us were hurt as children: we were mistreated, misled and, worse, mishandled. When abuse (verbal, physical, and/or sexual) happened to us, we had an immediate shift in our assumptions about the world. Specifically, for children who suffer abuse at the hands of a caretaker or a predatory stranger, safety and security has been eternally ruptured, and a belief in the benevolence of the world and its people is often too hard to achieve.

The unyielding result is that we grew up angry. And many of us are still angry. We are angry at the world. We feel and act like it owes us something. We hate everyone around us, and we hate ourselves for who and what we think we have become. Many of us who have survived child abuse divide the world into two types of people: Those who have been hurt, inappropriately touched, "affected," "singled out," and "damaged" versus those who were lucky enough to be safe, untouched, and therefore, unable to relate to us.

Like all other emotions, anger begins as a neurological response to our perception of specific events. As a result, many of the conclusions we draw from them will be erroneous. Additionally, anger can have a major impact on our inner world. This may manifest in physical sensations such as disruptions in sleep and appetite and even cognitive changes.[3] It can impact the choices we make regarding friends and lovers, and it can engender changes in our social life, prompting us to withdraw and isolate from others around us.

In order to understand anger's impact on your past and current choices, it might help to answer the following questions. This will allow you to focus on the source of your anger, as well as the patterns of behavior that have become your current mode of relating in the world. Remember, anger is a unique subjective experience that can promote feelings of guilt, shame, self-loathing, and depression. Thus, we ask:

Do you still hold onto a lot of anger and hatred in your life? Where do you think it stems from?

_____

_____

_____

_____

_____

Who are the people and what are the things you hold the most amount of anger and hatred toward and why? Take inventory.

_____

_____

_____

_____

_____

What are the reasons *you hold so much anger and hatred within you?*

_____

_____

_____

_____

_____

Now that you have identified and elaborated on some of the sources of your anger, as well as the ways you likely react to this emotional arousal, you are closer to being able to gain power over this arousal state. Self-examination, especially as it pertains to anger and hatred, can be a frightening experience. This is because the effort to understand our anger requires sacrifice and risk.

The sacrifice: The things we hold as true about ourselves (especially on a once-unconscious level) must be confronted and possibly surrendered. But when we confront the truth behind our anger, we discover that we are actually vulnerable, sometimes frightened, and even a bit helpless.

The risk: The feelings of anger that we explore must be experienced with our whole being. We will not succeed in healing our anger if we seek respite in denial or lies. Therefore, when we examine our inner world, we risk feeling uncomfortable, uncertain, and alone. We are forcing ourselves to face the contradictions in our life: We want to see ourselves as strong, but we fear we are weak. We want to make a change in the world, but we feel powerless to change anything. We discover that we have been betrayed, promises were broken, and lies were made to us. In the end, our faith is challenged.

Thus, anger can have a powerful effect on our spiritual development. Many will question our faith in religion, in God or a higher power. Other survivors of abuse will ask existential questions such as:[4] "What kind of God lets this happen to us?" The answer is unclear, and in the absence of any satisfactory answer, we lose spiritual faith, and we feel helpless.

What are the obstacles holding you back from having faith in a meaningful or purpose-filled world? What is your view on the presence of a higher power?

_____

_____

_____

_____

_____

_____

_____

It is a courageous task to hold onto our faith in the presence of ongoing trauma (be it trauma that is occurring in the present day, or trauma that recurs in the form of repetitive or compulsive flashbacks). Many of us lose faith in goodness, and when we are confronted with the question of our suffering, we become technologically minded, grounded in the here and now. This is where our attempts to conquer the evil thoughts and feelings that we have inside are met with failure. Specifically, we tell ourselves that we are committed to becoming *heroes* of our own fate, but we are doing so without the help of a spiritual affiliation, group support, or individual guidance. In the end, we find ourselves retreating, feeling defeated, and the cycle of self-hate and anger starts all over again.

This sense of defeat is known as **shadow anger**.[5] We have attempted to understand, and even accept, who we are, and what has happened to us, but we still have our demons to wrestle. It is thus necessary that we appreciate that shadow anger is indeed still a part of us. Our demons will not go away simply because we will them to. In fact, they become a part of our ego that, as psychoanalyst Carl Jung asserts, remain necessary for our survival. If we do not find healthy ways to express these thoughts and feelings they will likely fester or leak out in distorted or even dangerous ways. In psychology, this is called **covert hostility**, and it reflects an unconscious display of rage, or even violence, toward one another.[6]

Are you doing, or have you started to do, the inner work so you are able to understand your demons?

_____

_____

_____

_____

_____

_____

If the answer was yes, what have you begun to learn about yourself as you face these demons?

_____

_____

_____

_____

_____

_____

In attempting to answer these questions, you may have discovered that, like every one of us, you still have some more work to do. This is because anger, like nuclear waste, is nonbiodegradable.[7] It can be buried, but it will eventually leak and poison everything in its path (our health, our work, our relationships, and our belief systems). Thus, we must learn to express our anger mindfully, and with the ultimate goal of learning ways to let it go.

The active expression of mindful anger, in a safe and self-compassionate way, is a core component of sincere and successful healing. Thus, we attempt to preempt the simmering rage and resentment we have felt all too long on the inside by sharing it with someone (clergy, therapist, or friend) or by writing it in a journal to ourselves in a manner that can be heard, integrated, and considered.

Practice Mindful Anger

To reduce the struggle involved in this emotional experience, we recommend a cognitive behavioral technique called **mindful anger**. This is an exercise that individuals can use to help themselves to self-soothe in the midst of feelings of anger and hatred.

1. *Crisis: "What was done to me that caused my anger?"*

_____

_____

_____

_____

2. *Belief: "What is my immediate (and potentially impulsive) thought or belief?"*

_____

_____

_____

_____

3. *Alternative Belief: "What other interpretation can I consider about myself, or my abuser, at this moment?"*

_____

_____

_____

_____

This exercise, which utilizes the techniques of mindfulness and self-compassion, can help us reregulate our emotions during episodes of extreme arousal. The underlying principle at play here is an assumption that the crisis (abuse) was our fault (belief). But when we challenge these unconscious and erroneous beliefs by actively considering alternative interpretations of the event, we discover that the abuse was not our fault. Growing up scared caused us to develop survival strategies, such as false memories, erroneous interpretations, and adaptations in our thinking. Simply stated, in order to survive the pain, we told ourselves that the negative actions that were levelled against us were our fault entirely.

EXERCISE 2

Practice True Power

True power is born of integrity, and it has three antecedents:

1. The first is the ability to master control over our emotions, for if we lose control, we lose vision; and without vision, we have no internal power.[8] We admit that we have emotional vulnerabilities, and we recognize the different forms of self-destructive action that arise from having those feelings. We "name the monster" in our effort to "tame the monster." Instead of participating in our emotions, we observe, watch, and narrate what is happening to us, both physically and emotionally. How would you name the monster (demon) that lingers in your psyche?

Narrate what you observe of this demon as if he or she were a character in a movie or book.

_____

_____

_____

_____

_____

_____

_____

_____

_____

The Childhood Trauma Recovery Workbook for Adults

2. The second is the ability to **discern the mistakes of our past** from the potential successes of our future. In order to achieve this goal, we must be able to observe ourselves *without judgment*. This is the dialectic of our human condition; we are capable of acting badly at times, while we are still good people at our core. We are hurt, and we are still learning ways to deal with our overwhelming emotions, and are, thus, deserving of self-love and self-compassion.

Write down a few compassionate sentences to the inner child who needs your healing right now:

_____

_____

_____

_____

_____

_____

_____

_____

_____

_____

3. The third is **flexibility of view**. Think of people you may have punished for actions or behaviors that had little to do with them. Think back on what his or her truer intentions may have been. Recognize that your friend, partner, or mate is as human as you are, that he or she has needs and wants that are not always spoken about, or asked for, in effective or healthy ways. When you honor these truths about your well-intended friends, you are less likely to cut off or punish them for "being human like us." *Cut-off* acts like an immediate painkiller; it releases neurotransmitters called endorphins, and this helps us to heal a wound in the immediate moment. But the relief is only temporary, and we slowly, and remorsefully, discover the long-term cost and dangers of our impulsive need for vengeance and release.

What do you want to say to a friend or partner you may have yelled at, or hurt unjustly?

_____

_____

_____

_____

_____

_____

_____

_____

_____

_____

True power in a loving relationship means that we are not *threatened* by the words or actions of someone we love. Rather, we are compassionate toward the other's needs while we remain merciful *upon ourselves*. Self-regulation, vulnerability without judgment, and flexibility of thought will all help us to tame our feelings of anger and hatred.

Healing the angry self is achieved by allowing the monster to emerge in the context of a safe environment or loving relationship, as well as through constructive modes of expression. Through honest dialogue, we attempt to shine the light of consciousness into the darker places we were once afraid to explore. With love and acceptance from a partner, mate, or therapist, we find that our shadow self is not as scary as we had imagined. Specifically, once expressed and integrated, these fears can take their place as important markers on our path toward developing a healthier sense of self.

When we wrestle with the presence of anger and hatred in our lives, we discover ways to effectively "break up" with them. We sit beneath the shadow that these memories cast until we learn to embrace them and understand what they came here to teach; for they came here to teach us about *forgiveness*. Only once we manage to forgive ourselves for the things that were done *to* us, not *by* us, and only when we understand the true virtue in forgiving those who have hurt us the most, can we disempower the demons that once controlled us. We will suddenly see life in a new light—the light of mercy. But if we do not find forgiveness, we will repeat the cycle of anger and hatred.

Have you found forgiveness for yourself? If not, what would it take to do so?

_____

_____

_____

_____

_____

_____

_____

_____

_____

_____

Have you found forgiveness for those who hurt you the most? If not, what would it take to do so?

_____

_____

_____

_____

_____

_____

_____

_____

_____

_____

Of all the tasks that surviving child abuse has set before us, reaching a place of forgiveness is by far the hardest. For many of us, the word itself seems to carry within it the contents of an unfathomable goal. Indeed, thinking that we can (and even *must*) forgive what happened to us will undoubtedly be met with feelings of shock, disbelief, and a renewal of old anger. As survivors of abuse, we never asked for this job, and we feel unprepared and unwilling to do the necessary work.

Perhaps a more manageable approach to understanding the concept of forgiveness is to break the word down to its smaller parts. Looking at the word acrostically, we can surmise that each letter carries within it a different, but equally important, charge. More specifically, when we **forgive**, we:

Faithfully surrender to the possibility of a higher power

Overcome our wish for retribution or retaliation

Recognize that what was done to us *was not our fault*

Grieve the loss of our innocence and sense of safety for as long as we need

Invite others to share in our sorrow so we are not alone on this journey

Valiantly pray for the rehabilitation or repair of the one who hurt us

Educate the world about what we are learning

Whether we are mourning the loss of our innocence, wrestling with our anger and hatred, or struggling with the concept of forgiveness, we know that our journey will be difficult. But we also know that *success is possible*. We can grow and we can change. Some of us will re-experience moments of shock and disbelief, while others will feel the calm that comes from surrender. Some of us will challenge our identity, while others will discover roles and responsibilities we thought we would never have. Many of us will question our faith, and others among us may find a renewed love for our Creator. And through it all, the lessons we learn from wrestling with our anger and hatred will be our consolation, our bounty to work with, for the next part of our journey in life.

When you are ready, reach out to those who have hurt you the most and attempt to forgive them. It can be in the form of a letter, a prayer or thought, or even a face-to-face conversation. Afterward, feel the weight of your anger begin to lift from your shoulders.

The Childhood Trauma Recovery Workbook for Adults

You can use this space to start composing your thoughts.

_____

_____

_____

_____

_____

_____

_____

_____

_____

_____

Now allow yourself to rest. This is hard work, and it requires courage and strength. But it also requires self-love and self-compassion. You are growing as you read and work through every page of this workbook. Take a moment to praise yourself, for you are on your way to a new and healthier way of living.

2

Depression and Anxiety

In moments of weakness and distress it is good to tread closely in God's footsteps.

Alexandr Solzhenitsyn

From the first day that we suffer abuse, depression becomes a part of our everyday life. A mental health disorder, depression manifests as a persistent feeling of sadness, malaise, and loss, robbing us of energy, vigor, and interest in things we once found meaningful. It can devitalize our sense of power or control to the point where we are unable to work, to love, or to find purpose in our life. And if we suffered abuse as children, the alterations in our mood and our energy, as well as our self-image and our view of the world, all become part of a more chronic cycle of ups and downs.

Children who are depressed endure the specific pressures of academic stress as well as social isolation, bullying, and poor impulse control. Parents do not always understand the signs and symptoms of this disorder, and they may respond to a depressed child with unreasonably harsh punishments or low tolerance for what they perceive as abnormal. As depressed children we may have withdrawn emotionally, hiding our feelings of fear, shame, or dread from caretakers and friends. We have become physically unavailable, through hours of solo play in the bedroom (protracted periods of fantasy play with toy cars or action figures), or unabated episodes of gaming in a dark room on the computer.

In order to understand the impact depression had on your childhood and/or current life, it might help to answer the following question. This will allow you to identify and locate your memories and your responses to those memories. Remember, depression is an emotional experience that changes our self-image as well as the ways we view others in our world. Thus, we ask:

What signs and symptoms of emotional depression did (or do) you struggle with?

_____

_____

_____

_____

_____

For many survivors of abuse, depression reveals itself through a range of negative physical symptoms as well, including changes in sleep patterns (we find ourselves either sleeping all day or we are unable to sleep at all) and alterations in appetite, energy level, and immune function.[9] Specifically, when we are depressed, we are at greater risk for glandular disruptions (changes in digestive flow in the stomach or colon) and immune system breakdown (vulnerability to host diseases such as ulcerative colitis or Crohn's disease), and we lack the self-concern or strength to maintain proper physical self-care. Remember, depression is also a physical experience that changes the functions in our body. Thus, we ask:

What signs of physical depression did (or do you) struggle with?

_____

_____

_____

_____

Depression also underlies many addictive and compulsive behaviors, such as alcohol and substance abuse, stimulant craving, overspending, hypersexuality, gambling, and even addiction to love. Anatomically, the body's normal regulation is responding to the abuse we suffered through **chronic hyper-arousal**.[10] If our body was hurt by an abuser, we grew up experiencing an unanticipated "jolt" to our nervous system. Now, as adult survivors, we find ourselves seeking out alternatives to this original "jolt," only this time at our own doing. This is our body's way of "regulating" our internal emotional world. Simply stated, the reckless or impulsive actions we take become our negative, albeit adaptive, attempts at obliterating the pain we feel deep inside.

What actions and behaviors did (do you) participate in to either numb, reenact, or challenge the arousal states of depression in your body?

_____

_____

_____

_____

_____

A fundamental goal in your ability to manage reckless actions is to find the healthy balance between your rational brain and your emotional brain.[11] This balance helps you maintain greater control over your decisions. Take a few slow, deep breaths now, and you will find that your heart rate will decrease and your body will begin to calm down. As you take these breaths, pay attention to each inhalation and each exhalation. Notice how the oxygen is nourishing your body and helping you to return to a more balanced and rational state of being.

Review of Depression: Signs and Symptoms

- **Persistent low mood:** an overwhelming drop in mood from a previously normal state.
- **Reduced energy:** psychomotor retardation manifested through episodes of extreme fatigue, malaise, and "slow-motion" activity.
- **Loss of interest in usual activities:** hobbies become more like chores, work becomes overwhelming and uninspiring, friendship feels tedious and tiring.
- **Poor concentration:** planning behaviors are disrupted, heightened distractibility and low attention to the task at hand.
- **Disruptions in memory:** wavering in certainty and detail of a past event. This is related to a 12 percent reduction in the size of the hippocampus (memory center of the brain) due to cortisol toxicity.[12]
- **Changes in sleep:** inability to fall asleep (insomnia) or overlong episodes of sleeping (hyper-somnolence). Some psychiatrists include chronic episodes of "early morning awakening" as another sign of endogenous depression.

- **Changes in appetite:** unexplained weight loss due disinterest in food, or dramatic weight gain as a result of using food for self-soothing.
- **Anhedonia (absence of pleasure or reward):** an inability to enjoy, savor, or appreciate the gratifications of life. Loss of a sense of inner reward.
- **Rage/irritability:** outbursts of anger that are often incongruous to content; pressing urge to pace about, fidget, or remain "in flight."
- **Nightmares:** the unconscious feelings of fear, sorrow, or dread that are expressed during sleep.
- **Withdrawal:** removal of self from ordinary activities and attachments.
- **Feelings of helplessness:** an inability to effect change in the world; this includes a reflexive and immediate rejection of suggestions or techniques to improve one's condition or situation.
- **Increase in mood-altering behaviors:** misguided efforts at self-medication and self-regulation using illegal substances, alcohol, spending, sex, and gambling.
- **Cognitive distortions:** Brief, disorganized thoughts about reality that are invulnerable to logical feedback from friends and family. This might include "catastrophizing," or magnifying the importance of small mistakes that were made.
- **Spiritual alienation:** disengagement or estrangement from a belief in a higher power or a universal force that once grounded a person's particular belief system.
- **Self-loathing:** negative, self-abasing statements and feelings that reflect critical opinions of self. This usually generates from erroneous feelings of self-blame for things that were done *to* us, and not *by* us.
- **Suicidal ideation and urges:** profoundly altered perception of ourselves and of the world around us characterized by feelings of defeat, worthlessness, and self-destructive thoughts and wishes.

It is important to note that not every depressed person will experience all these feelings. Depressive symptoms can be idiosyncratic to specific personalities, and they vary according to family history, genetics, the types of support networks that are available, the age of the child at the time of abuse, and other varying life events. We offer the checklist above so that you can locate and identify whether any (or many) of these symptoms sound familiar to your own personal experience. If you recognize yourself in some of the above, reach out to a good friend, clergy, or therapist, as this can be a good start toward healing.

Additionally, utilizing the following exercise can aid in ameliorating some of the malaise and helplessness you may feel during your depression.

Structure Building

To reduce the malaise, self-doubt, and disorganization induced by depression, we recommend a cognitive behavioral technique called **structure building**. This is an exercise that individuals use to create greater order in their day. The underlying tenet here is that *structure helps us to regulate our affect*. Simply stated, when we engage in activity, our mood usually lifts. In addition, upon completion of a structured activity, we feel a sense of mastery and accomplishment, two emotions that help generate positivity in our sense of self.

Structure building is a three-step process that includes:

1. Creating the day's schedule in such a way that all tasks are written, by hand, on a piece of lined paper. Writing tasks down stimulates the prefrontal cortex in the brain, a part of our mental engine known for activity, direction, and control. The tasks we write down are called **targets**, and they consist of any activity, from brushing one's teeth and taking a shower to picking up the mail and paying the bills. Once a target event is completed, the next one is already waiting on the list to be accomplished. The schedule should be written in one-hour increments, allowing time for well-earned breaks and rest.

2. Each day's schedule must contain one target event that involves self-care. This can be a visit to the gym, or a walk outside or in nature. Even if your movement is limited, or you have never exercised before, there is always a physical fitness move that you can do that remains within your safety limits. Physical fitness tasks stimulate the impulse conduction of dopamine, which is a neurotransmitter in our brain stem that promotes feelings of happiness and well-being. In addition, norepinephrine, a neurotransmitter that helps regulate energy and mood, is also released through exercise and contact with nature.

3. Each day's schedule must also contain one target event that involves helping another who is in greater need that we are. Known in dialectical behavior therapy (DBT) as "doing what's effective," this target event creates a lift in emotion and energy through the abetting of someone else's unfortunate problem or situation.[13] It redirects us back to our inherent loving energy, which is an inner force that overrides our temptation to

judge others, and ourselves, negatively. It forces us to use the spirit of self-discipline to hear the voice of compassion for ourself and for others, and it effectively silences the voice of the hurting ego that once told us that we were unworthy.

The thirteenth-century Persian poet Rumi once said,

> *Travel through life as a pawn travels, one slow move at a*
> *time, to redeem the wide-ranging nobility of the queen.*

This beautiful poem suggests that every one of us holds merit and grandeur through our inner loving nature, and by going at our own pace. But those of us who were abused at a young age have learned to anesthetize our pain. We believed the words we were told by unkind caretakers or predatory strangers when they called us "unworthy," "incompetent," or "good for nothing." Thus, *structure building* acts as an immediate release from the isolation and blunted affect we learned to adopt as hurt children. It frees us to act in effective ways and to recognize that others are in need, just like we are. And it helps us to remember who we are when we are at our best.

Now that you have learned healthy and effective ways to empower yourself through momentary episodes of depression, try answering the following questions:

What tools do you have in place to help you deal with your depression?

_____

_____

_____

_____

_____

_____

Are you in any form of talk therapy, such as cognitive behavioral, psychodynamic, dialectical behavior therapy, existential, trauma, or grief therapy? If yes, how has the therapy helped you to gain greater understanding of your depression?

_____

_____

_____

_____

_____

The psychological problems that arise from child abuse not only render us vulnerable to depression, but also to anxiety. Sometimes considered a sister disorder to depression, anxiety manifests itself through the activation of our traumatic memories, and we often struggle with effective ways to manage them. Rather than feeling a sense of power and connection, the abusive event(s) create a rift in our core assumptions about the world and its people. The result is that we are left with feelings of disempowerment and disconnection from others.[14] We have undergone life-threatening events, psychic or bodily assault, or the crossing of sexual boundaries, and our sense of safety, and mortality, have been altered.

Acknowledging that anxiety is a true feature of our present mental state is an *integral sign of our strength*. It takes initiative and courage for us to admit that we are anxious and afraid, for we are telling the world, and ourselves, that we are no longer passive. Far from granting victory to our abuser, we are taking action to foster our recovery. The ability to feel a sense of mastery and control over our abuse takes precedence over all other things. And we can achieve this successfully when we are willing to place vulnerability and trust in a safe and secure relationship with a therapist or wise friend.

When did your anxiety first set in, and do you know why?

_____

_____

_____

_____

_____

Anxiety resulting from early abuse causes us to lose trust in others, and it stunts our ability to emancipate into independent and confident adults. We thus approach adult tasks with the burdens of lowered ability for self-care, poor organization, confusions in identity, and an inability to form stable and lasting relationships. But the telling of our story, in all its gory details, to someone who is willing and able to listen to us, is how we heal from the anxiety that once kept us down.[15]

Who have you told your story of abuse to? How did the telling of your story effect your healing journey? If you have not yet told your story of abuse to anyone, perhaps you can use the space below to begin the narrative.

_____

_____

_____

_____

_____

_____

_____

EXERCISE 4

Tell Your Story

When you are ready and your relationship with your therapist or healthy friend feels safe and secure, you may wish to tell the story of what happened to you. There are four healing components to the telling of our story, and they are the following:

1. We gain mastery and control over our anxiety.

Those of us who have been exposed to trauma in childhood are left with feelings of disempowerment. We feel weak and untrusting of others. This is because, at an innocent age, we were swept into a world of unpredictability and the expectation of recurring danger. Our belief in justice and mercy was challenged, and we came to learn that, sometimes, bad things happen to good people. Thus, the recounting of our story helps us to own the anxiety. We gain control over the crisis, and we achieve power over what happened to us and to our family. "This is my story," we tell ourselves. And the more we tell it, the more we understand about this new and strange world we were thrown into.

2. We accept what happened without silencing or minimizing.

Well-meaning friends rarely allow us the freedom to express the despair we feel over our abuse. We know that our life has been changed forever, but our friends and family search for our return to our "lighter" selves. They define our healing through our actions of happiness, and they naively offer us affirmations of hope. But these words do not soothe the hearts of those of us who were hurt by life.

"Time will help you heal."
"God only gives us what we can handle."
"It's time to move on."

These are the well-intentioned words of friends who want to fix what they perceive as broken within us. But they do not know that it is not their job to fix anything. Thus, when a good listener hears our story, details and all, we feel safe because our vulnerability is being honored. And vulnerability in the context of a loving connection is where our healing begins.

3. We integrate the traumatic event into memory.

Neurophysiology research reveals that abuse in childhood (and other traumatizing events) is processed differently in our brain from normative and/or common events.[16] Whereas common memories become blended and remain accessible to our awareness, traumatic memories are not integrated into our hippocampus (memory center). Thus, the memories remain separate, and partially or fully out of our consciousness. As a result, we who are survivors of child abuse are at risk for suffering from **disruptions in memory**. It is as if our brains were too scared or shocked to be able to make sense of the horrors we went through. But when we tell our story to someone who truly understands us, we light up the memory center in our brain.

4. We "place" the memory alongside our developing sense of self.

The more we tell our story of hurt, the more we "place" it somewhere where it no longer defines us. As victims of childhood trauma, we worked diligently at hiding our pain and we rarely, if ever, processed these negative memories. Instead, we became adept at denial, minimizing or secretly owning our story as the sole definition of our selfhood. But we are now ready to be heard. But when someone finally hears our story, they can ask us the following questions:

"Do you remember a place in that story where you were strong, even heroic?"

"How did you manage to get to safety?"

"Were you aware of a personal or inner strength deep inside of you?"

When we "place" our traumatic memory, we move it from "front and center" to a place beside us where it quietly remains. Unbidden and unwelcome, our story is only a part of us now. Not the whole of us. We can now begin to see ourselves with compassion and forgiveness. We are no longer victims. We are victorious, for we have survived and are working hard to live a better life.

EXERCISE 5

Perform a Ritual Event

Researchers and psychologists who study abuse and trauma in childhood suggest that the process of "placing" our pain somewhere where it no longer defines us is successfully facilitated through performing a ritual event.[17] Ritual events include:

- Writing a letter to your abuser. You can say everything you never had the courage to say. Then you can burn the letter, bury it, or read it to a trusted friend.
- Throw away an item of clothing that reminds you of the time you were hurt.
- Paint your feelings on a ceramic plate, put it in a cloth bag, and then smash it in a safe manner, or run over it with your car.

Ritual events help us to "place our grief" in a symbolic fashion. For some, this exercise will generate a sense of relief when performed, while for others, it may stimulate, temporarily, more memories and more sorrow. Regardless of how our ritual event moves us, the act of "placing" our pain will eventually help us to live "alongside" our fear and our sadness, and not to live "behind or beneath them."

Now that you have gained greater appreciation of the ways depression and anxiety impact your daily functioning, you are ready to create your own list of tools and strategies for greater self-care:

Emotional Self-Care: *Write down a list of ways that you can care for yourself when you are depressed or anxious (e.g., meditate, create a structured list of target events to complete, tell your story to a friend).*

_____

_____

_____

_____

Physical Self-Care: *Write down a list of ways you can care for yourself physically when you are depressed or anxious (e.g., exercise, massage, soft music, long walks in nature, connect with others).*

_____

_____

_____

_____

Spiritual Self-Care: *How do you care for your spiritual self (e.g., prayer, poetry, scripture, reaching out to clergy, watching a sunset)?*

_____

_____

_____

_____

If our story of abuse or fear is not handled carefully, it can become the new and sole definition of who we are. "I am a victim," or "I am different because I was raped as a child," we hear ourselves say. While self-expression is indeed essential for healing, we all need to eventually integrate our trauma into a larger, healthier sense of self. We are all more than the sum of our most frightening memories. Eventually, our statements of who we are *becoming*, not just who we *were*, are the medium through which we successfully develop a healthier self-image. "Becoming" involves the actualization of our inner gifts, our self-pride, and our determination to succeed in this life. Thus, we stand taller and with greater pride, for we are no longer afraid.

The focus of this chapter has been to help you gain greater appreciation of how depression and anxiety have been impacting your path to healing. With recognition and awareness comes understanding. And with understanding comes relief. As you grow into a healthier, more self-loving adult, you will recognize how your self-image is changing. Where once it was held hostage by someone else's selfish acts, now it is expanding and allowing you to identify your strengths. Remember, if you are reading this workbook, you are a survivor. You contain hidden strengths within you that helped you to make it to where you are today. Praise yourself for being who you are. And bless yourself for who you are *becoming*.

3

Grooming, Lies, and Manipulation

Ordinary riches can be stolen, real riches cannot. In your soul are infinitely precious things that cannot be taken from you.

Oscar Wilde

I n 1653, Guiseppe Francesco Borri, an Italian physician and alchemist, gained infamy as a self-proclaimed "seer" for people with afflictions and maladies. He achieved this status by claiming that the Archangel Michael appeared to him in a dream and bestowed upon him the ability to see into other peoples' souls. So charismatic was Borri that wherever he went he attracted followers for his fabricated visions. Princes and merchants flocked to consult with him; and, in 1662, the Amsterdam Magistrates conferred upon him an honorary citizenship.

But Borri was never able to "see" into other peoples' souls. What Francesco Borri saw were peoples' *wishes*, their emotional vulnerability, and their repressed needs. Like all false messiahs, Borri was masterful at mirroring the wishes of his followers, and he promised them things that were otherworldly, magical, and *external*. This is the nature of the abuser: He will claim the gift of understanding and compassion, and gradually set himself up as a source of authority, attention, and love. But after the bond has been created, this seemingly ordinary relationship is profoundly disrupted.

This is known as grooming, and the process is insidiously carried out by means of forced secrecy, manipulation, and lies. The targeted child is unaware of the pathological attachment that is developing. He or she has little knowledge that this "trusting" connection is actually the abuser's way of seducing, exploiting, and dominating his or her world.

The characteristic behaviors of control and violence have an innocuous beginning, and the actions of the abuser may look innocent at first, manifested as small statements of disapproval where the child is made to feel responsible for things he did not do. Eventually, the overtures strengthen and include an erratic enforcement of rules; the child is rewarded for doing something that pleases the abuser, and then punished for having competing relationships in their life.

Abusers select their target through assessing the ease of the child's accessibility, as well as through their perception of his or her vulnerability. Harmless discussions become more and more intense, and sometimes this leads to sexualization. For example, hugging or tickling eventually escalate to increasingly intimate dialogues and acts of physical contact, such as massages or showering together. The attempt to make this behavior seem natural and acceptable in the eyes of the vulnerable child is always paramount in the process.

Eventually the child discovers that they are unable to escape the predatory actions, and they adopt a position of learned helplessness. This is known as **adaptation**, and it requires an internal state of hypervigilance, or constant alertness.[18] The child quickly learns to recognize potential warning signs, such as changes in the abuser's facial expression, voice, body language, mood, and level of intoxication. This nonverbal communication becomes automatic, and sometimes occurs on an unconscious level.

If the offender is well-known or highly regarded in the community, they become easy to trust and follow. An overwhelming sense of helplessness develops in the child, which only serves to strengthen the maladaptive attachment to the abuser. An energy of terror mixed with love ultimately develops, and the child will sacrifice his or her own welfare to maintain this bond.

The Six Stages of the Grooming Process

1. **Targeting the Child:** The perpetrator will carefully observe a child in an effort to detect their weaknesses, including, isolation, loneliness, neglect, a disorganized family life, or lack of parental supervision.

2. **Trust Building:** Perpetrators make deliberate efforts to gain the trust of parents or caretakers of the child.[19] These actions abet the process of gaining more access to the

child as they are providing seemingly kind attention. At this stage, the offender will collect important facts about the child, such as his favorite games and television shows, and they will find ways to fill those needs.

3. **Developing Status:** Once the perpetrator begins to fill the child's needs, he gains greater emotional and physical status in the child's life. This will manifest through the giving of gifts, flattering the child, offering money, and meeting the basic needs of food and warmth to ensure the effectiveness of the traumatic bond.

4. **Separating the Child:** The perpetrator attempts to segregate or sequester the child by creating situations in which they are alone together (tutoring, coaching, or babysitting). The perpetrator will then reinforce the trauma bond through telling the child that he loves and understands the child in a way that others, even parents, do not.

5. **Eroticizing the Relationship:** Once dependence and trust have been built, the perpetrator will gradually sexualize the relationship.[20] This takes the form of showing pictures joking, teasing, and creating situations in which both are naked (swimming or showering). The adult exploits the child's naive curiosity and uses physical stimulation to progressively eroticize the attachment.

6. **Manipulation and Control:** Once the abuse is occurring, the perpetrator will make threats to maintain the child's participation and continued silence. The offender will manipulate the child into keeping everything a secret, and he will blame the victim for "wanting this all along." Most importantly, he will convince the child that the loss of this "special relationship," or the consequences of exposing it, will be too much of a risk for the child to survive.

In Their Own Words

The contributions in this section are from child and adult veterans who have experienced abuse firsthand. It may be difficult to hear or read some of the excerpts that follow, but we believe that bearing witness to the stories of others has a healing component. *Story as medicine* is a technique used in many healing traditions.[21] It is based upon the premise that every one of us has feelings and fears that are awaiting attention and affection. And if we are brave enough to read, or listen to, the testimonies of others who have been where we once were, we will discover outcast parts of ourselves—the parts we thought we successfully buried. More importantly, we will recognize the parts of our inner core that still remain sacred and intact.

Targeting: In recounting the grooming behaviors that one survivor endured, we learn the damaging effect of being the target of an abuser. The following account describes how, at the age of eight, this survivor was carefully targeted among other children who were around him:

> My abuser had been watching me all day at the public pool. He saw that I spent a lot of time alone away from others, and that he would have easy access to me. I spent the afternoon exhausting myself, running around, jumping in and out of the pool, mostly alone. I think the pool closed at six o'clock, and everybody began to disappear. It was time to get home. I grabbed my things and headed to the changing rooms. I had no idea that my abuser had followed me in there—and that's when it happened.

Trust Building: Discussions about child abuse are made difficult because they evoke fear and discomfort in the listener.[22] These fears are exacerbated by media headlines and internet news reports that highlight the child abuser as a "monster," a "pervert," or a "dangerous stranger." But research reveals that more often than not, the perpetrator lives within the walls of the child's house, or is that "cool Uncle" or friend of the family. As a result, the grooming becomes even more insidious, as friends and family watch seemingly "healthy" interactions go on right before their unsuspecting eyes. In the words of one survivor:

> He would walk up to me at the bus stop, put his arm around me, and walk off with me in front of my friends, telling me that this is what I want. Looking back now, when I ask my friends what they thought about that man in those days, they all said they figured he was a friend of my parents who came to bring me home from school.

Developing Status: A fantasy attachment relationship begins to develop where a child thinks his needs for warmth and nurturance are being met. Family and close friends may fail to recognize the maladaptive relationship and instead spend more time focusing on the child's immediate behaviors, such as poor school performance, irritability, or disruptions in sleep or conduct. But quietly germinating beneath the surface is a trauma bond that is virulently growing. In the words of one adult survivor:

> He gifted me a toy car, told me I was beautiful, and he would come and watch me play soccer and told me that I was the best little soccer player on my team. One time he said, "Look at you turning into a big boy now.... into a handsome young man."

Separating: Abuse presents a child with a dilemma or "double bind" when it comes to remaining connected to the outside world. If a child maintains close connections with his "normal" world, he is at risk for telling someone about what is happening. If he or she does speak up, the abuse will end but the consequences will begin. Telling someone may create a rift in the family, and the actions of the offender, to whom he or she has grown attached, may cause him to go to prison. These conflictual thoughts help cultivate a belief that it is safer to say nothing, and remain isolated. In the words of an adult survivor:

> I was made to believe that no one understood, loved, and accepted me like my abuser did. This resulted in my belief that I had to distance myself from friends and family, eventually to be forced to cross emotional, physical, and sexual boundaries. I thought I felt love for this man. I thought I was in a relationship with him.

Eroticizing the Relationship: When an emotional attachment and sufficient separation have been established, the perpetrator attempts to erotocize the bond. In the words of one survivor:

> He repeatedly told me how special I was, that he loves me and I love him. He sexualized the relationship and I began to believe that this is what I wanted. There was no getting out of it; he was the one I trusted and thought I loved.

Manipulation and Control: Many survivors recount the recurring fear of danger in their stories. The child is often forced into silence through the threat of death. Sometimes the child is warned that fighting back, or telling the police, will end in violence toward or murder of someone in their family, even perhaps a beloved pet. Firsthand testimony from a survivor of rape described:

> The first words he said to me were that if I told anyone, he would kill me and kill my family. He told me that I will get in trouble with the police if I ever say anything to anyone. He told me that people thought I was a liar and that everyone hated me. He said he was the only one I could trust—the only person who liked me and would take care of me. Otherwise, I would be all alone.

EXERCISE 6

Debriefing

After having reviewed the stages of the grooming process and read the testimonials of some survivors, it is not uncommon to find yourself experiencing feelings of discomfort.

The Childhood Trauma Recovery Workbook for Adults

This is known as **re-traumatization**, and it happens because the stories of others can sometimes provoke memories and emotions that you may have thought you put away.

Take a moment to focus on what feelings or emotions have been stirred in you. Use the space below to write them down. Remember: When you have the presence of mind to know that you are struggling, you also have the ability to place those struggles somewhere where they can no longer hurt you. This is known as **trauma debriefing***, and it is a good way to release the feelings that have been aroused in you.*

_____

_____

_____

_____

_____

_____

_____

_____

_____

_____

The great American poet David Whyte once wrote:

> *Those who will not slip beneath*
> *the still surface on the well of grief,*
>
> *turning down through its black water*
> *to the place we cannot breathe,*
>
> *will never know the source from which we drink.*

This poem describes the power that trauma debriefing can have in our healing process. Specifically, when we feel dark and overwhelmed, we tell our story. We write it down or express it through prayer, believing there is a force that transcends our understanding and has our ultimate healing in mind. We march forward with faith, and we come to discover that we will, eventually, be healed. Yes, our heart is aching, but our soul is growing. We are becoming wiser and healthier versions of ourselves.

The next part of this chapter is devoted to several other symptoms of grooming, lies, and manipulation. They include Stockholm syndrome and trauma bonding.

Stockholm Syndrome

Stockholm syndrome is a coping mechanism that reflects the strangely positive emotional attachment a hostage feels toward his or her captor or abuser. The victim develops changes in the view of the world that he once knew and a psychological connection between the two develops. Secretly, a victim of abuse begins to believe the offender is actually a loving friend.

The condition was first named in 1973 by a Swedish criminologist named Nils Bejerot, who studied the behaviors of survivors of a Stockholm bank robbery. During a six-day stand-off with police, many of the bank employees expressed feelings of sympathy toward the robbers. Some even refused to testify against their captors in court; a select few raised monies to help support the captors in their defense.

Signs and Symptoms of Stockholm Syndrome

- Feelings of affinity toward the offender
- Identifying with the beliefs and behaviors of the offender
- Negative feelings toward law enforcement or other authority figures
- Flashbacks
- Lack of trust in an ordered world[23]
- Inability to maintain calm
- Heightened startle response

The cause of this condition has several key features:

1. **Being in an emotionally charged situation** for a protracted amount of time, a dependency upon the hostage-taker develops. The basic needs for food, water, and shelter slowly embed themselves into the dynamic of the relationship. When these needs are met, a neurological system of positive reinforcement takes root.

2. **Sharing a space with an abuser**, especially when conditions are poor (not enough food, physically uncomfortable or tight quarters) can create a feeling of a "common

struggle." "The enemy of my enemy is my friend," the captive tells himself. "We are in this together."

3. **When threats to a hostage's life are not carried out**, an insidious belief that the captor is interested in his victim's ultimate welfare develops. This belief becomes more prominent if the captor does not dehumanize the victim.

4. **Learning to surrender to the will of the captor** secures a victim's safety. Over time, the victim may even feel a sense of gratitude to his captor and view him as humane.

Have you suffered through any form of grooming, lies, and manipulation that eventually led to Stockholm syndrome? If yes, what was it like for you?

_____

_____

_____

_____

_____

_____

_____

Trauma Bonding

Another negative effect of child manipulation and exploitation is trauma bonding, which is a deep connection that develops between a victim and abuser. Similar to Stockholm syndrome, child victims can develop feelings of love and fidelity for their abuser. Warmth and affection are basic needs of childhood, and children and teens face the greatest risk falling into a trauma bond. In the words of trauma researcher and author Beverly James, children, like heat-seeking missiles, will find warmth and caring where they can.[24] The attachment that develops is a *fantasy relationship*, but it offers, at times, moments of attention and care when a hurt child needs it most.

Children who are exposed to sexual exploitation and targeted grooming are the most likely to develop a trauma bond. Some may have never experienced physical intimacy; thus, the grooming tactics of the offender can lead a child to believe that the abuser has genuine feelings of love and concern for his or her welfare.

Signs and Symptoms of Trauma Bonding

1. **The victim refuses help or support from family members, friends, or professionals who work in the field of child safety.** Moreover, the victim will avoid everyday family activities, choosing rather to sequester themselves to their room or to spend time with friends that are nameless, remote, and hidden from the family.

2. **There are sudden behavioral changes and changes in personality.** A child who was once social and confident will suddenly appear sullen, secretive, and withdrawn.

3. **They will come home wearing new clothes, jewelry, or watches that they clearly did not buy for themselves.** This is the most common form of grooming, and it facilitates the trauma bond.

4. **The victim will defend the abuser once the truth has been found out.** This may include surreptitious meetings with the perpetrator even after the relationship has been sanctioned and forbidden.

5. **The victim will resist moving on from their abuser.** New friends and healthy (age-appropriate) activities will be shunned and sworn off by the child.

The formation of trauma bonding has several key factors:

1. **Promises and tokens of affection are given to the child in an attempt to manipulate the trust and loyalty of the unsuspecting child.**

2. **The child will be suspicious of authority figures who can help: This reflects the victim's erroneous belief that the abuser can protect them from danger.** This is common in child trafficking cases, as a victim fears physical harm from myriad potential abusers.

3. **The victim is influenced to break away from family attachments.** This is the abuser's manipulative way of isolating the victim as a means of greater control and power.

4. **Learned helplessness sets in.** This is a belief that there is no escape from the abuser. The victim preconsciously believes "I'm damned if I do and damned if I don't." This psychological phenomenon becomes a precursor to depression in the child, and it helps the victim to identify with the aggressor.

The trauma bond is solidified slowly and strengthens over the course of time. The hurt child is more focused on *short-term survival* than the *long-term repercussions*. Surrender thus becomes an immediate act, a plea for "instant peace" rather than the possibility of "long-term war."

The Childhood Trauma Recovery Workbook for Adults

As part of your healing process, you may find it helpful to take an inventory of a person (or people) who have exploited you in this way. Do you still have any form of relationship with them today? If the answer is yes, what is the quality of this attachment?

_____

_____

_____

_____

_____

_____

Trauma Bonding in Adulthood

Trauma bonding in adult relationships manifests in a cycle of love and hate that is sometimes referred to as **veneration** and **denigration**. We idealize our partner at first, and then come to hate him or her as time passes. But still we remain in the relationship, unconsciously acting out old familiar patterns of this love–hate cycle. The degree to which we reenact these old patterns is strikingly high. This is because emotional themes from our abusive past are always threatening to resurface, especially when egos are clashing.[25]

The cycle of veneration and denigration plays out as follows: We see our partner as "all-knowing" and capable of great things. Then, he or she disappoints us. We fight, sometimes with rigor, always needing to have the last word. Then, we relent and find ourselves surrendering to a deeper need for peace and acceptance. It is at times of surrender that we entertain a range of excuses as to why we allow this behavior to continue. These may include statements such as:

- He'll change. Give him time.
- He didn't really mean all those things he said.
- Maybe she was right, I *was* out of control. It *was* my fault after all.

One of the reasons we allow these behaviors to persist is known as **gaslighting**. Gaslighting is a form of emotional abuse that causes us to doubt our own actions, and ultimately, our own sanity.

It can involve subtle tactics of manipulation that are employed by a partner, such as constant criticism, lies, and escalation of denial.[26] (Denying our feelings, memories, and even our reality.)

Have you been in an adult relationship where the cycle of veneration and denigration has occurred? If the answer is yes, how did you regain clarity and greater confidence to stand in your own truth?

_____

_____

_____

_____

_____

_____

What tools and techniques have you put into place to ensure this does not happen in future relationships?

_____

_____

_____

_____

_____

_____

The purpose of this chapter was to introduce you to the methods of manipulation and grooming that are used by unkind adults to influence and overpower young and impressionable people. In reviewing this information, you will find yourself, at times, feeling tired, sad, or even overwhelmed.

But please remember, there is a reparative function to the work that you are doing. In hauling up old memories and feelings, you are giving yourself the chance to finally place them somewhere where they cannot hurt you. Those who undertake the journey to heal from the abuses of the past come back carrying medicine for us all.

This leads to freedom.

4

Impostor Syndrome and Self-Sabotage

Make yourself a door in which to be hospitable, even to the stranger in you.

David Whyte

If you could speak to your childhood self, what would you tell him or her? For most of us, the healthy answer is "It wasn't my fault!" But those of us who have been traumatized in our youth live out our adult lives with an unrelenting belief that we *were* to blame for our abuse. We were the recipients of manipulation and lies and, in our attempt to understand what was happening to us, we accepted those lies and manipulations. Confronted with our memories in later years, we either challenge their veracity, or we deny their place in our history.

Some of us anesthetize ourselves from the pain of these projected lies by using substances, sex, gambling, and love. We tell ourselves that our abuser was correct, that we do not deserve joy and peace, and we end up sabotaging all the good in our lives. One of the causes of this self-sabotage is known as **impostor syndrome**, and it is an unconscious defense mechanism that many of us employ to stave off, or avert, the pain of our youth.

Simply stated, when we are hurt as children, our identity is mortally challenged and we *accept* our abuser's projections of us as bad or unworthy people. We *become,* in our minds, whom and what the abuser expected or wanted us to become.

While the *Diagnostic and Statistical Manual of Mental Disorders (DSM-5)* does not recognize impostor syndrome as a mental health disorder, it is a common occurrence, particularly in people who have experienced a trauma or life-threatening event. It is characterized by an unrealistically negative assessment of our competence and our skills.[27] Specifically, it is difficult for us to accept praise; we would rather berate ourselves or our performance rather than believe the positive words of others. In more extreme circumstances, we may even handicap ourselves by engaging in behaviors that sabotage our chances for success. In the most extreme cases, impostor syndrome can lead us to engage in potentially dangerous or reckless activity.

Review of Impostor Syndrome: Signs and Symptoms

- **Negative Self-Talk:** The inner critic that consciously or unconsciously warns us of our limitations and failures (e.g., "I can never do anything right." "I'll never amount to anything in life.").

- **Cognitive Distortions:** Patterns of thinking or believing that involve inaccurate or erroneous interpretations about ourselves or the events happening around us.[28] Originally coined by psychologist Aaron Beck in 1960, it is commonly linked to stress, anxiety, and depression.

- **Black-and-White Thinking:** A rigid cognitive style where words such as "always" and "never" are overused; sometimes manifested in alternatively idealizing and devaluing people.

- **Rebuking the Positive:** Tendency to view positive events as "flukes" or aberrations. (A common disqualifying statement is "Yes, but...")

- **Over-Personalization (Taking the Blame):** Blaming ourselves for things over which we have little or no control. This also takes the form of feeling responsible for other people's struggles.

- **Minimizing and/or Magnifying:** Placing stronger emphasis on negative events and downplaying positive ones.[29]

- **Should and "Why" Statements:** A rigid perception of rule following, usually taking the form of self-imposed expectations. The words "should" and "why" almost always provoke in us a sense of guilt and/or shame.

- **Perfectionism:** A trauma response that urges us to believe we must be absolutely perfect or we will be "found out" as unlovable or unworthy.

- **Overly Independent:** A proclivity to disqualify the help or support of others since that would make us feel like we are not capable of success on our own.
- **Over-Setting Goals:** Reaching for improbable outcomes and feeling disappointed when we fall short of them.

A simpler way to understand the underlying energy at play in someone who struggles with impostor syndrome is to consider it a defense mechanism. What is involved here is that we are defending ourselves from a painful inner conflict—a conflict about our true identity.

"Am I as competent, worthy, and good a person as I *think* I am?" we ask ourselves, "Or am I, like my abuser told me, a bad person who wanted this abuse?"

In projecting, or *adding*, our "positive" features onto other people, we are successfully disavowing, or *subtracting*, them from our own subjective experience. This creates a reduction of our inner conflict. Our abuser's words are still in our head, and through an unconscious memory, they are forcing us to feel and behave in ways that are congruent with *their* fantasies and feelings about us. It is a type of *psychological coercion*, coming down from the voice of the abuser, verifying our *erroneous* assumptions about ourselves.[30]

What motivates a child to collude with his or her abuser in this way? What causes us to believe things that are simply *not true*?

One answer is our desire for love and validation. Our actions, as children, are motivated by a need for love, acceptance, and guidance: We need to be cared for. This primitive need creates a strong tendency in us to *accept* our abuser's projections. Then we *identify* with their expectations. The real truth is that our abuser hated *him or herself,* and he or she placed this unacceptable emotion onto *us*.

"You think I am unworthy, then it must be true," we tell ourselves.

In this way, we become a collusive participant in our abuser's hidden agenda. This is in full effect throughout our dependent years of childhood, but especially at the nodal point of the abuser's coercion, manipulation, and grooming.[31] This is how the process of our identity formation as "bad and undeserving people" rapidly accelerated.

Have you, or do you now, live with impostor syndrome? If yes, what are some of your symptoms?

_____

_____

_____

_____

_____

Have you done the therapeutic work necessary to understand, and even find peace, with the trauma you suffered? If yes, what have you learned from doing this work?

_____

_____

_____

_____

_____

_____

"What Is a Part of Me" vs. "What Is Definitely *Not* a Part of Me"

To better help you return the erroneous, negative statements you were told about yourself as a child, we ask you to gently confront your own denied feelings of self-worth. Close your eyes and try to get as comfortable as possible. Breath in through your nose and out through your mouth.

Now, imagine yourself as the embodiment of the powerful, competent adult you were originally born to become. See yourself as that person.

What do you sound like?

_____

_____

_____

_____

_____

How do you walk?

_____

_____

_____

_____

_____

How do you dress?

_____

_____

_____

_____

_____

What are the positive features that other people envy about you?

_____

_____

_____

_____

_____

_____

This exercise will be difficult at first, since those of us who were hurt as children were taught to believe the negative things that were said about us. But take your time. Breathe. And imagine yourself at your personal best. Envision the beautiful adult that your higher power planned for you to become. Think about how you will change the world.

Now, write down what you envisioned in the space below. These can be simple statements that begin with the words "I am..."

_____

_____

_____

_____

_____

_____

The second part of this exercise is to *carefully* envision the negative or horrible features that existed in the person who hurt you. Identify these aspects in him or her, and understand that every one of those negative features was erroneously projected (transferred) onto you when you were young.[32] These awful feelings existed inside of the abuser, *not* inside of you. They were *never* a part of you.

Now subtract these features from your inner view. They do not belong there anymore. They were placed there, coercively, by a predator who was once shamed into believing these negative things about themself. *Subtract* them from your personal database and *add* them (*return them*) to the person who wrongfully gave them to you.

Continue to breathe deeply...and naturally...as you gently release the negative features in your database that never belonged there.

Now, write down what you envisioned in the space below. These can be short statements that begin with the words "I am NOT..."

_____

_____

_____

_____

_____

_____

Exercises such as these can be exhausting, as they ask us to haul up thoughts and feelings from deep within. Some of us have long buried these feelings. Others of us have denied they were ever there. This is good place to stop your reading and take a break. Get in touch with the elements of nature, for that is how the dopamine in your brain will regenerate and calm you.[33] If you cannot go outside, do something that enhances your spirit. Listen to music, focus on a sunset through your kitchen window, or watch a favorite television show. Now is the time to care for yourself. You are getting stronger with every exercise but, as with a hard workout in the gym, you may find that you are tired, emotionally sore, and in need of rest.

. . . .

The next part of this chapter is devoted to understanding a similar symptom of trauma, namely **self-sabotage**. Sometimes considered a sister disorder to impostor syndrome, self-sabotage occurs when we hurt ourselves physically, emotionally, or spiritually, thereby hindering our own success. We become quite good at undermining our goals and silencing our inner values. The literature regarding trauma responses in children is replete with references to this form of activity. In the aggregate, these studies define self-sabotage as a form of **dysregulation of emotion**, and it is used, like all other defenses, in the service of surviving our inner pain.

More specifically, children who are trapped in an abusive environment are most likely forced to tolerate their pain. Faced with this formidable task, they search for ways to preserve a sense of trust in a world that is otherwise perilous and untrustworthy. They create new methods of controlling a situation that is terrifying and unpredictable. But the only means of coping that are truly available to hurt children are immature or underdeveloped psychological defenses.

Simply stated, abused children adapt through developing "habits of the hurt."[34]

One of these habits is to **identify with our aggressor**. The children establish a **trauma bond** with the aggressor in order to survive. As discussed in the previous chapter, a trauma bond is a set of internal expectations that children develop about upcoming interactions with the abusive adult. Because they are unable to prevent the abuse, they form ways to placate the abuser, or act in a manner that the abuser will find acceptable. This is how hurt children survive. They focus on the needs, wants, and emotional mood of the abusive adult in order to maintain safety for themselves.

The most common form of placating the abuser is known as **automatic compliance**.[35] Because the abuse causes children to feel high levels of anxiety, they are more likely to miss many cues, or they will block out stimuli that could enhance their understanding of the situation. As a result, children eventually learn to express complete and unwavering obedience, and they shut off from their **wise mind**. The term wise mind comes from dialectical behavior therapy research and practice, and it denotes the part of our thought processes that are regulated by reason and logic rather than emotion and impulse.

This is the development of the defense mechanism known as self-sabotage. The remnants of the past have depleted our self-confidence and they compel us to create negative or self-defeating habits that serve to protect us from the pain of failure. Normal or rational fears (those connected to ordinary events) are now out of balance; they confuse us, and hold us back from succeeding in our careers and our relationships.

Review of Self-Sabotage: Signs and Symptoms

- Choosing a partner who is incompatible
- Refusing to fully commit to a relationship
- Unrealistic expectations of others
- Chronic mistrust
- Over-criticizing friends
- Holding grudges
- Silencing the self (not speaking up for one's own need)
- Procrastinating at work

The Childhood Trauma Recovery Workbook for Adults

- Disorganization
- Inability to make decisions

As seen above, the origins of our feelings of powerlessness can toxically play themselves out in our adult relationships, and in our work. But we can change the trajectory of the trauma; we can discover new ways to trust and to relate with others. We do this by transforming or deactivating old credos, for they no longer serve us. Thus, we learn to refer to ourselves with positive words.

Say It Positively

We all carry an internal narrative within ourselves, sometimes without our awareness. It is the inner voice that all too often criticizes or challenges our sense of competence and worth. Those of us who struggled with our self-image as children are more likely to focus on preconceived notions that we are not good enough, or that we are destined to fail. Through these internal dialogues, we deceive ourselves into thinking things that are simply not true.

Positive self-talk is our attempt to change the narrative. It helps us to switch the automatic assumptions we have about ourselves. We catch ourselves in the middle of our unconscious negative scripts, and we flip the valence. This has a proactive effect on our feelings and ultimate actions.

In the following space, write down the automatic negative statements that you likely say to yourself.

_____

_____

_____

_____

_____

_____

Now take each negative statement and proactively switch it to the positive. Before you begin, place your hand over your heart and feel yourself breathe. Imagine that your heart is like a closed-petalled flower that, with your kind words, is opening gradually to the warmth of the sun.

_____

_____

_____

_____

_____

_____

This exercise was designed to help you discover the loving and compassionate phrases that you needed and deserved to hear when you were young and afraid. The automatic negative words that you replaced with positive phrases can become a mantra. You can rewrite them as many times as you need. You may want to turn them into wishes, or prayers. You can say them out loud or whisper them to the child inside of you.

Honor the positive words and sentiments that you are discovering about yourself. And if you notice that your mind wanders and veers to the negative, you can refresh your statements by taking a deep breath, and trying the positive again.

The Triad of Self-Love

This exercise is designed to help you locate and identify the features inside of you that are worthy of love and validation. It involves three tasks that are to be completed in order.

1. *Make an inventory of your greatness. Ask yourself, "Who am I when I am at my best?" This includes the moments when you were most proud of yourself. Write these moments down in the space below:*

_____

_____

_____

_____

_____

_____

2. *Make a list of three people who are your **private audience**. These are the people in your life who have always believed in you. They are the ones who know and love you just the way you are. It may be a beloved grandmother, parent, therapist, coach, or teacher. It can be a person who is alive, or someone who has passed away but stays with you always in spirit. Your personal audience is always with you, especially when you are feeling low and think you have lost your way. Write down the three people who are in your private audience:*

_____

_____

_____

3. *Name one person whose life is better simply because you loved him or her. For every one of us, there is a person in this world who is better because we were in their life. This may be a friend who has your number stored in their emergency speed dial list, ready to be pressed if they were ever in trouble. It may be the child you sat with at the edge of the sidewalk who cried because he could not find his mother or father. It may be the child inside of you who needs your adult love and nurturance. Write down the name of that person here, for somewhere, someone needs you:*

Our use of words can either harm us or heal us. The last two exercises have been designed to help you notice, more clearly, the words you say to yourself, and to others. Acclaimed essayist and author Susan Sontag refers to words as inhabiting wisdom:

> *Words mean. Words point. They are arrows. Arrows stuck in the rough hide of reality.... They resemble rooms and tunnels. They can expand, or cave in.*

Understood in this way, the words we choose create spaces that can be inhabited, re-settled or re-colonized. What we say to ourselves can imbue emotional conflict, hate, and shame. Or it can inspire love, acceptance, and the realities of rapture.

Now that you have read through this chapter, studied the concepts and constructs of impostor syndrome and self-sabotage, and practiced the exercises designed to strengthen your sense of self-love and acceptance, we ask you to answer the most important question of all. If you could speak to your childhood self at the time you were abused or traumatized, what would you tell him or her, and why?

Have you accepted the true power that you hold inside of you? Do you embody this power? Do you live it every day? If not, what do you think you need to reach a place of greater acceptance for who you truly are as a lovable and worthy person?

_____

_____

_____

_____

_____

Of all the tasks that trauma has set before us, reaching a place of acceptance is by far the hardest. Indeed, thinking that we must accept ourselves, shame and all, can leave us angry, despairing, or feeling hopeless. But do not despair. The day is long and there is still more work to be done. Follow through to the completion of this workbook. Healing takes time. And you are indeed healing.

5

Shame and Ego

You can close your eyes to reality, but not to memories.

Stanislaw Lem

Shame is a debilitating force, or energy, that exists within every one of us. It is experienced as a compelling and advising voice that emanates *from inside,* and it is the genesis of many of our self-defeating and self-destructive behaviors. Shame has roots in "attachment theory."[36] Specifically, feelings of a healthy attachment to a caretaker give rise to a sense that we are loved—we are safe and secure and we know that we belong to someone who will care for us. For most of us, this is our mother or father, and they become the orienting figure(s) in our life. The "good" parent is the *home base* from which we learn to confidently branch out into the world.

It is in this first love relationship that we develop a template, or pattern, for how to behave in all other loving connections. It is also the place from which our sense of self is born. If we were raised by a parent who was physically and emotionally available to us, we developed feelings of worthiness and self-love: "If my needs are being met without struggle," we say to ourselves unconsciously, "I must be deserving of the love I receive."

But children who were raised in abusive environments often respond as if they have disturbed attachments patterns; they demonstrate feelings of self-loathing and secret shame. Lonely, self-doubting, and sometimes hateful of others, hurt children keep these emotions close to the chest. The abusive relationship becomes a pattern of relating fearfully to others; old visions and memories of danger, hurt, and loss can be resurrected in new attachments.[37] Like anesthetic to pain, hurt children hide from exposing themselves to others. But anesthesia eventually wears off, and when it does, the scared child comes to discover the hold that shame has had on him or her all along.

"If you knew me, the *real* me," we whisper under our breath, "you would feel differently about me."

Of all the intrusive and unbidden thoughts and feelings trauma survivors experience, the most dominant one is shame. This emotion is less amenable to change than other behaviors from stress and trauma. But understanding the signs and symptoms of shame can ultimately help us to locate, identify, and name the impact that shame has on our everyday lives. And when we identify our shame-related behaviors, we can be more successful at changing them.

Review of Shame: Signs and Symptoms

- **Feelings of Self-Hatred:** Feelings of disgust with oneself or one's body. It can lead to self-sabotage as was discussed in the previous chapter.

- **Self-Destructive Behaviors:** Thoughts or actions of self-harm such as cutting, burning, binge eating, and purging. It can also manifest in reckless acts of unprotected sex, driving while intoxicated, extreme sports, drug and alcohol abuse, and criminal activity.

- **Reenactment of Abuse:** Choosing partners or friends who remind us of the abuser. It can involve choosing friends or partners who have similar mannerisms, speech patterns, or style of dress of the abuser.

- **Modeling the Abuser's Behavior:** A pattern of acting like, or taking on the qualities of, the person who hurt us. We discharge our shame by treating others we love the way our abuser treated us.[38]

- **Self-Neglect:** Not providing ourselves with the basic needs of proper nutrition, clothing, sleep, or safe shelter.

- **Isolation:** Remaining "cut-off" or remote from others. This is often motivated by an unconscious belief that we will not be hurt if we stay alone, hidden, or withdrawn. This also manifests in an inability to strike up conversations with others in public situations.

- **Self-Critical Tendencies:** Being harsher with ourselves than we should be; being unforgiving of small mistakes we may make.

- **Perfectionism:** An attempt to avoid being further shamed by never making mistakes.

- **People-Pleasing Actions:** Feeling over-responsible for other people's happiness. It manifests as a need to put on a false-front; we attempt to portray ourselves as more confident than we really feel. This derives from a wish to avoid further shaming.

- **Lack of Motivation:** Inability to follow through with goals or tasks. Sometimes it manifests in an inability to commit to a career path or to a partner.
- **High Tolerance for Mistreatment:** A pattern of allowing partners and friends to mistreat or abuse us.

High Tolerance for Mistreatment

This is perhaps the most commonly undetected symptom of shame in survivors of abuse. We often find ourselves in bad relationships and ask ourselves:

"Why do I continue to let people hurt me?"

We entertain a range of excuses as to why we allow this behavior to persist. These may include statements such as:

"When he's bad he's bad, but when he's good he is sooo good."

"Give it time, she'll change"

"He loves me, I know it. He just has a strange way of showing it."

"Maybe I deserved that treatment; after all, nobody's perfect."

Family therapists and psychology researchers alike have long studied the answers to this difficult issue. The findings range from psychoanalytic interpretations, all the way to behavioral learning theory. We offer a neurochemical model of shame adaptation here:

Each of us contains something akin to a pharmaceutical storehouse in our brains. One group of chemicals, known as endogenous opioids, ignite during moments of intense fear and trauma. Thus, when we experience an abuse in childhood, opioids begin to surge and create a post-traumatic stress response.[39] As we grow older and move further away from that trauma, the opioid system diminishes in our brain, and we go through a withdrawal, not unlike drug withdrawal.

Then we meet someone who unconsciously mirrors the person who once hurt us. Suddenly, our unconscious brain is activated, *triggered* by negatively charged memories from our youth. (These triggers are particularly stimulated to the senses of smell and sound.) At these moments, there is a reacceleration of the opioid system in the brain; and we find ourselves "feeling that familiar feeling." We are at once drawn to the (neurochemical) charge we receive by the person or the event. While we know the negative charge is bad for us, our brain is telling us that it is *familiar*. And "familiar" is what draws us ever-nearer to repeated episodes of hurt and danger.

Recognizing and Naming Our Emotions

Learning how to *recognize* our emotions is the first step in being able to *name* them. And when we *name* the emotion, we can *tame* that emotion. This way we gain a healthier control over our feelings.

Most of us do not pay close enough attention to the way other people make us feel. We spend even less time focusing on how people inspire us to act, or "react." Thus, the following exercise is designed to help you examine yourself in front of people who make you anxious or create a sense of emotional urgency. The goal is to learn how to notice your triggers and listen to them as possible warning *signs*. This will allow for ways of making healthier decisions.

Pay attention to the physical changes in your body:

How does this person make you feel *inside*? Try to identify the physiological sensations as they occur in this person's presence. This may include muscle tension, butterflies in the stomach, or the hot rush of panic filling the chest cavity or shoulders. These are the triggers that are talking to you through your body. They are here to guide you, not to hurt you. Remember, our bodies never lie. They tell us things we may not always want to hear. But they never lie.

What is *your* body telling you?

1. Identify your immediate urges:

This is your chance to describe how your physical sensations made you *want to react*. Identifying and labeling feeling states (especially feelings of threat), known as "enhancing emotional awareness," will ultimately help you to modulate *how you react*. Using this technique, you will eventually experience a reduction in anxiety symptoms.[40]

Did you feel a strange, familiar, pull as a result of these physical triggers?

_____

_____

_____

_____

_____

_____

Did you have an urge to know this person better?

_____

_____

_____

_____

_____

_____

Did you want to say or do something drastic, risky, or even dangerous?

_____

_____

_____

_____

_____

_____

Remember, *urges are only impulses driven by thought*. They are *not* facts; rather, they are your body's arousal system alerting you to something. Once you *identify* the sudden urges you feel, give them a name.

"I feel *tingly* inside."

"My shoulders feel *hot and tight*."

"My chest is *burning* with a rush of heat."

After naming the feeling, it is necessary to put a space between that feeling and your actions.[41] You will discover that there is indeed a difference between what you want *to do at that moment, and what you* actually *do. This is a sign of growth and a cause for hope. Use the space below to write these feelings down:*

_____

_____

_____

_____

_____

_____

2. Assess and allow the feelings to exist.

After the event is over, it is important that you review the situation in detail. This is your opportunity to process the longer-term consequences of your decisions. If the experience was distressing, make a list of the pros and cons of tolerating your healthy action. The goal of this part of the exercise is to understand that some distress in life is unavoidable.

Pros:

_____

_____

_____

_____

_____

_____

Cons:

_____

_____

_____

_____

_____

_____

Please remember that the distress you feel is a part of the process of changing and getting better. In order to ultimately experience *positive* feelings, you must first allow for *negative* feelings. This is how you move *through* the pain to a place of greater comfort.

――――――――――――――――― EXERCISE 11 ―――――――――――――――――

Find Your Voice

One of the most common reasons for patients to attend therapy is to "find a voice" so they can speak up in ways that allow them to be heard, and ultimately, validated. As mentioned earlier, many of us feel as if we have lost the courage or safety to share our feelings. Shame has robbed us of our vigor and confidence; we have learned that it is easier *not* to speak up.

This style of relating can create trouble in our adult years, for if we rarely, or never, express our more authentic feelings of anger or hurt, we will become vulnerable to releasing them in unproductive, and even dangerous, ways. Specifically, thoughts or feelings that are avoided run the risk of leaking out like toxic waste. Unprocessed and unexpressed, they remain where they are, threatening to emerge as physical symptoms, such as backaches, stomach problems, or disruptions in sleep and appetite, as well as emotional malaise and embittered interactions with loved ones.

If we speak our peace, and not our war, we will release ourselves from potential discord in our future relationships. In so doing, we will come to discover that our words are as important as those of our friends, coworkers, and mate.

Use the space below to write down a feeling or an opinion that you have been afraid to share with someone important to you. This is your opportunity to find the voice of the child inside who was silenced by fear, doubt, or shame. You can write something simple or you can write something of great depth. The idea is to release the thoughts and feelings that have been buried deep within.

Shame closed the door on your ability to speak your peace. Confidence will now reopen that door. Your feelings, and your words, *matter.*

_____

_____

_____

_____

_____

_____

Life has a way of forcing us to grow, even under the most uncomfortable conditions. For the soul will not rest until its essence is revealed. Thus, we cry out. We cry out in therapy, or we cry out to a close friend who loves and understands us. We give voice to our distress; we speak openly about our once-hidden shame. And if we are fortunate enough to find a listener who can hear us in all of our vulnerability, we will heal, for we are finally being accepted for who we are.

Crying out is not a weakness. It is a strength. It is a flexing muscle deep within the hurting soul that says "Find me, heal me, value me." And when our cry is met in a generous and understanding way, we begin to consider the possibility that we are *indeed* worthy. Through this prayerful benediction (and loving acceptance), our feelings of shame, self-doubt, and self-hate are released from captivity. And we move from a place of being entrapped to being embraced.

Give yourself a chance to share what is inside of *your* solitude, *your* shame, and *your* secret.

And learn what it feels like to be embraced.

Do you love and accept yourself for everything you are? If not, use this space below to be heard. Say or write down the feelings of shame that you have been holding too close to your chest.

_____

_____

_____

_____

_____

In writing down your feelings above, you have given yourself a chance to share what is inside of *your* solitude, *your* shame, and *your* secret. Imagine that someone you trust is reading the words you just wrote down. Imagine that special someone honoring your story, and loving you, *because* of your struggle.

This is what it feels like to be embraced.

. . . .

The next part of this chapter is devoted to understanding a similar construct to shame, namely ego. Much has been written about the ego, beginning with the seminal writings of Dr. Sigmund Freud. According to Freud, the ego is the part of the mind that mediates between conscious and unconscious desires. It is a metaphysical energy that forms the basic foundation of identity.[42] Simply stated, the ego is the unconscious part of us that facilitates the way we think about ourselves.

The word "ego" has taken on a related, but different, meaning. Specifically, in colloquial speech, the word is defined as a feeling of being superior to others. It reflects a person's sense of self-importance, and it is considered to be the root of our arrogance or overgrown pride.

In the aggregate, both definitions guide us to understand the ego as the core of the "self." But children who have suffered trauma or abuse never had the luxury of knowing an authentic self. They have been taught to hide or disown their thoughts, feelings, wishes, and desires. Left undetected and unable to express themselves clearly and safely, hurt children are less capable of identifying and respecting their uniqueness.[43] They have muted their senses and run from their inner world, and their egos are constructed through fantasy and make-believe.

Shakti Gawain, the internationally renowned teacher of consciousness, once said profoundly:

> *Everything in the Universe, including every part of ourselves, wants love and acceptance. Anything [inside] that we do not accept, will simply make trouble for us until we make peace with it.*

The powerful image behind this quote is that our own personal healing from abuse is dependent upon finding ways to understand and accept the authentic ego inside of us. She asserts that we all have a *shadow* to explore—a shadow that contains feelings and thoughts that have been rejected, repressed, or disowned. If we do not work to recover, and ultimately embrace, these cut-off parts of our ego, we will grow to manifest the opposite energy; namely, we will develop an overgrown, inflated, ego, filled with arrogance and false power, in an attempt to stave off the shame it really feels deep inside.

Write a list of when your ego took over a situation. How did these actions make you feel?

_____

_____

_____

_____

_____

_____

You may notice that the actions or behaviors you listed above were generated from a deeper place of fear, desperation, or a lack of confidence in yourself. This is because, in the absence of self-confidence, we act out our rage against the ones who love us.

We are all human. And we are all, in one way or another, hurt humans. Some of us are afraid of getting too close to another person. Some of us are easily frustrated because we hunger for an intimacy that we feel we may never find, or do not deserve. And some of us are afraid to simply talk about who we really are—to say out loud "This is what I need from you."

What are some things that you are afraid to share with another?

_____

_____

_____

_____

_____

_____

Reclaim Your Power

Now is the time to discover the source of your power and how you can tap into it. Paradoxically, power comes from failure, depression, and loss.[44] More specifically, when we are confronted with feelings of despair, we are being challenged to find the will to persist and rise again. Power's crucial foundation is the ability to wrestle with, and ultimately master, our emotions. But most of us search for power and confidence in outside places. We think that by building muscle in the gym, or wearing expensive clothing, we will feel powerful and confident. This is not true, for confidence comes from *within*. It is born of our own inherent qualities. It has been inside of us all along.

This exercise is designed to help you reclaim the power and the confidence that is inside of you. The prompts that follow are intended to help you wrestle with feelings of failure so that you can ultimately show up as victorious.

1. Remember a time when you allowed yourself to cry in the presence of another person. If you were fortunate enough to have revealed your insecurities to a caring and compassionate soul, you learned that your trembling, and your sorrow, were followed by insight, knowledge, and understanding. There was a revelation that came with a feeling of love and connection. The breakdown became a breakthrough; and, instead of shrinking from the shame you were forced to carry inside, you were, for just a moment, full and tall with the vision of how your loving friend saw you.

2. *Ask yourself: What does it mean to be vulnerable? For many of us, the very sound of the word "vulnerable" summons feelings of weakness. But in nature, we see signs that are quite the opposite. For example, a reed, or stalk of tall grass, is more powerful than a cedar tree, for the reed can bend beneath the storm without breaking. This metaphor teaches us that when we are soft, we are strong; we can take the blows that fate has thrown at us without snapping. We are still here, and we are growing every day.*

_____

_____

_____

_____

_____

_____

_____

3. Know the meaning of the expression: "The prisoner cannot free himself."[45] When we suffer, we feel like nobody else knows our pain. It is like we are in solitary confinement, alone behind a locked door. But religion, philosophy, and even science have taught us that when we grieve, we need the compassion of someone else to open that door for us. We ask for help from another, and a turning point occurs.[46] We discover new ways of mastering our pain and sorrow. We learn that other people have felt similar to the way we are feeling now. Moreover, we see that *they* made it through their long nights of darkness, and now they can teach us the way to our own successful future.

4. Reconcile with the higher power inside.[47] When we grieve the loss of our innocence and safety, we turn inward toward our highest selves, and to our deepest faith. We admit to the existence of a force that is beyond our cognitive understanding. We carry on with faith, and we uncover who we are and what we hold most sacred. Yes, we are confused and despairing, but we are also capable of experiencing meaning and dignity in our lives. Surrender teaches us about strength, fortitude, and the will to move on, for we know we are never truly alone.

The struggle with shame and ego ultimately ends when we take ownership of everything we are: All of it—the good *and* the bad. We search for ways to express these feelings, and we recognize that none of us are perfect. But when we tell someone who loves us that we are hurting, we allow the shadow inside of us to emerge. Through honest dialogue, we attempt to shine the light of consciousness into the darker places we were once afraid to explore. With love and acceptance from our friends or mate, we may come to find that our shadow self is not as scary as we had imagined. Moreover, once expressed, accepted, and integrated, our shame and ego will take their place as important markers on our path toward developing a healthier sense of self.

6

Toxic Masculinity

The man who dies with the most toys wins.

Bumper sticker

G etting to know and understand ourselves better is a central part of the healing process, especially for those of us who were raised in abusive or traumatic homes. Child abuse in our early years gives rise to overwhelming and out-of-control emotions, which in turn create feelings of self-loathing, shame, and guilt. Our sense of personal power, and our feelings of control, have been muted, and our self-soothing techniques, even by the most heroic among us, have been mocked and vanquished.

As a result, many survivors go through life struggling with what they believe to be the stereotypical demands of their gender. These demands, or pressures, are placed on them through culture, society, religion, generational codes, and myths. In this chapter we will discuss the myth of the "masculine mystique." We believe this will be useful for male, female, and nonbinary readers, as we all struggle together to understand the pressures that impact our friends and loved ones.

Our civilization's history is filled with stories of male veneration. Men strive to tame nature. Men are hunters and fighters. Men leave their mark on all that they possess and conquer. As a result, boys grow up comparing themselves to other boys, and they all too often find themselves lacking, or falling short of, the hypermasculine attitude and mannerisms that they think are reflective of a "real man."

This hypermasculine display can become so excessive that some boys grow up to embody exaggerated ideas and attitudes about manhood. These ideas, erroneous from their inception, infiltrate men's ability to work, or to enjoy friends and family, as they are frantically searching for ways to keep up with the demands of society's wrong beliefs about them. In the end, men become overprogrammed in the art of seduction, competition, and control. But these ideas cripple their efforts to express a true, authentic sense of self.

Academic and popular writing now consider these traditional stereotypes to be toxic as they normalize violence, aggression, bullying, homophobia, and misogyny. "Toxic masculinity" as a term itself is not a condemnation of men or male attributes. Rather, it is a construct that places emphasis on the harmful effects that adherence to traditional male gender roles has on mental and physical well-being. Specifically, when boys and men feel uncomfortable expressing their emotions, and are expected to be stoic and self-reliant, all-powerful, and ever-victorious, stigma and shame develop deep inside.

In our effort to survive the pain of our abuse, we project the opposite emotions outward. We use manipulative and controlling strategies to help us feel safe and strong. We act tough and rugged. We watch how we walk and how other men speak. We are grown boys longing for the chance to be our truest selves. But some of us lost the fight, and we have turned our need for power and control into a false version of who we really are. And one day, we look in the mirror only to discover a masculine identity that, sadly, reminds us of our abuser.

Toxic masculinity is a disease. It has generated inequities of power in relationships, been the cause of violence against women, and shaped sexual relations, politics, and cultural norms. Sadly, it has also weakened the cohesiveness of families who are trying to remain open and tolerant of changing values and mores. Below is a list of signs and symptoms that you should be aware of.

Review of Toxic Masculinity: Signs and Symptoms

- **Acting Tough:** Believing men should be physically strong and emotionally stoic, even callous. Believing that behaviorally, men should be aggressive and in control.
- **Anti-Feminine:** Rejecting of all things that are considered to be "feminine." This includes crying, admitting to pain or loneliness, or asking for help.
- **Power:** Obtaining power through financial and social status.
- **Physical Prowess:** Believing men should push themselves to extreme physical limits, that even when injured, men "muscle through" the pain. Thus, visiting a doctor is seen as weak.

- **Rigid Gender Roles:** Believing boys should not be taught to cook, clean house, or take care of younger siblings.
- **Physical Attractiveness:** Believing it is not possible to be successful if a man does not look good.
- **Risky Behaviors:** Heavy drinking, tobacco use, extreme sports, driving fast-driving cars, engaging in unprotected sex.
- **Hypersexuality:** Never saying no to sex. Multiple sex partners is seen as acceptable.
- **Self-Restricting:** Being less likely to console a victim or intervene in a conflict if one's reputation might be compromised.
- **Control over Partner:** Telling their mate what they can and cannot wear, and who they are allowed, or not allowed, to talk to.
- **Critical of Other Men:** Harboring negative opinions about men who express their feelings openly.
- **Self-Sufficient:** Not likely to attend psychotherapy if they are struggling with mental health issues. Comments such as "Man up" and "muscle through" the pain, or "Men don't cry," are commonly used against men who wish to explore their inner feelings.
- **Homophobia:** Fear, hatred, or discomfort with people who are lesbian, gay, or bisexual.
- **Transphobia:** Criticizing other men who are attracted to, or are in relationships with, trans women.
- **Ready to Fight:** Expected to act strong, fight back when pushed, and never say no to a brawl.

The Cycle of Unmanageability

The toxically masculine man is secretly caught between two worlds: an outer world of confidence and bravado, and an inner world of shame and despair. His goal is to keep his secret from affecting his public persona. But eventually, the consequences come: unmasked lies, broken promises, excuses and apologies that lack integrity and heart.

Do you now, or have you ever, felt like you were living in two worlds? What were secrets about your sense of masculinity that you were trying to hide?

_____

_____

_____

_____

_____

_____

Toxically masculine men move from seemingly healthy relationships to sudden isolation, and this occurs in repetitive, predictable cycles. The cycles start with an isolating belief system containing false credos and myths, like "Real men are tough and I am not tough." It continues with a preoccupation of this erroneous belief as the man fights outwardly against it. Hypersexuality, toughness, risky behavior, and control of his partner are the outward manifestations of this inner fear.

Appearing like a "real man" has become the primary goal; it is the source of his relief, and the remedy for the pain he feels deep inside. But friends and family begin to challenge these behaviors, and this confirms his faulty beliefs about himself. Eventually despair sets in, and his only recourse is to isolate once again.

Recovery from this cycle involves a reversal of the isolation that has become his common mode of action. Paradoxically, men must allow themselves to experience moments of vulnerability, support, and intimate connection with another. It is through tolerating the distress and discomfort that comes from intimacy with one person that men can finally begin to heal.

In order to help you heal from your false credos and beliefs about masculinity, it will help to answer the following questions. This will allow you to focus on the source of your beliefs, as well as the patterns of behavior that have been, or still are, a part of your mode of relating in the world. Remember, toxic masculinity is the outgrowth of men having been groomed into thinking that vulnerability is bad, and not "manly." Thus, we ask:

What is masculinity to you?

_____

_____

_____

_____

_____

When was the last time you cried, and why?

_____

_____

_____

_____

_____

How did crying make you feel?

_____

_____

_____

_____

_____

You may have answered this last question with a negative statement, and this is okay. Crying makes many of us uncomfortable. This is because, when we share our feelings of sorrow with someone who cares, we are immediately pulled out of the secret world we were once living in. Now, expressed and exposed, we fear we will be judged, rejected, or worse, abandoned for our truer feelings. We have relied on false beliefs to guide us for so many years. But now, as we learn to cry with others, we can begin to let their love guide us the rest of the way. This is how we find our heroes.

The Path of the Hero

Many of us search for heroes in our effort to understand and become men. We need fathers to model for us, and then bless us; we need buddies to challenge us and share our coming-of-age stories with; and we need leaders to inspire us and to show us the way.

We are all too familiar with the myths, folklore, and religious stories of male leadership: Jonah finding his way in the belly of the whale, King David spying on Bathsheba from his rooftop, and Orpheus's death-defying trek to the Underground. These "anointed" men devoted their lives to fighting off shame, hostile competition, and the threat of annihilation. Thus, in our search for our own manhood, we too try to take the path of the hero, for we think that our hero will be the source of all our wisdom, masculinity, and strength.

We learn from all these tales and stories that, before he is permitted to achieve victory, the hero must renounce his boyish qualities. This includes his fear of humiliation, his desire for glory, and his struggle with loneliness. He must be willing to give up his life for what he believes in.

But this is *not* how a hero is born, for the path to manhood is not found through traveling *outward*, but from turning *inward* and finding the potential that exists there. All heroes are required to know their *inner* self while maintaining an authentic awareness of their outer presentation. For in stepping out of the pack, the hero works hard to understand and embrace his inner fears and insecurities. The truth is, in our attempt to understand manhood, the hero that we are really searching for already exists within each of us. He is emotionally expressive, has female friends and mentors, encourages compassion and kindness in others, listens and validates other people's feelings and needs, respects his mother and father for their sacrifices, and does not shy away from struggle or sorrow.

The Childhood Trauma Recovery Workbook for Adults

Who is your hero, and why?

_____

_____

_____

_____

_____

Now that you have identified the characteristics of your hero, what are the features inside of you that make you a hero in someone else's life?

_____

_____

_____

_____

_____

Think about someone in your life who looks up to you. This can be a younger sibling, your son or daughter, your beloved nephew or niece, or a student or patient that you teach and mentor. How does he or she see you?

_____

_____

_____

_____

_____

Now write down a list of the things that this child sees that you secretly disagree with. Then write down why you disagree.

_____

_____

_____

_____

_____

_____

Now, use the space below to challenge those statements. If you wrote: "My nephew thinks I have all the answers; he sees me as strong and powerful;" but you *secretly think* he is wrong, *challenge that secret impulse.* Remember, perception is reality in the eyes of those who love us. Maybe, just maybe, *he* is right and *you* are wrong. See yourself as your beloved children and students see you. With their image in your head, write down "Maybe I am..." (how that child sees me).

Maybe I am _____

Maybe I am _____

Maybe I am _____

EXERCISE 13

Cementing Bonds

The myth that men need to pull back from emotional displays of affection with friends needs to be reassessed.[48] This means that we must challenge societal norms and create new ways of relating to one another. This exercise is designed to help you establish a bond with someone you may have wanted to get closer to but feared the consequences.

1. **Cementing bonds requires that we make room in our lives for reflection.** This may mean attending a therapy session or a house of worship. It may mean getting in touch with the elements of nature, or setting time aside to be quiet and thoughtful. Uncomfortable

feelings may surface, for self-reflection stimulates feelings of anger, hatred, or other negative thoughts and memories.

2. **Think of someone in your current life whom you believe has the heart and the fortitude to hear your story.** This may be a trusted counselor or therapist, a family member, or a wise and beloved friend.

3. **When you are ready, make that call or send that text.** This is your opportunity to reach out to that person and begin the process of healing through sharing your truth.

4. **Breathe.** Take back your power. And share with this person your darkest secret. Openly communicate the pain, and break the stigma that "real men don't cry." A recent study on the tears we shed from shame, anger, hatred, sorrow, and depression revealed that there are enough toxins and poisons in these tears to kill a rat. Think about that...think about what it does to us when we hold those tears inside.

5. **Tolerate the discomfort that may come from having revealed your secret.** Think about how you trust this person to hold your truth. Remember that you chose them to carry the burden, the secret, with and for you. Honor this decision. It was a good one.

6. **Pay close attention to the muscles in your body, as they may be tightening or seizing up with fear.** If you are feeling tension in these areas, breathe it away. Tell yourself, "I am safe and secure in this trusting bond."

7. **Wait for their reply.** Hold onto the knowledge that you are changing. You are breaking the silence that once bound you to your abuser. You are bringing light to a part of your life that no longer needs to remain in darkness.

8. **Accept what comes next, for you will experience a kindness and an appreciation that will surprise you.** Perhaps for the first time in your life you will discover what it feels like to be heard. To be truly heard. This is love. This is the divine flow of acceptance and validation that you rarely, if ever, received when you were young and so in need of support.

9. **Embrace this moment.** You are cementing bonds. You are learning how to share. And you are discovering that you are not alone. You are never alone.

10. **Remember: it is okay not to be okay.** This is vulnerability.

American monk and spiritual writer Thomas Moore once said that, "The dreaming soul hears the voice of a true friend and, suddenly, the meaning of the word love is revealed."

And Rumi, the Persian poet, stated, "To a man dying of thirst, a friend is a cup of spring water."

So, here's to friendship. May your cup overflow with love.

. . . .

In this chapter we have reviewed the origin, as well as signs and symptoms, of toxic masculinity. We have discussed how hypermasculinity can become so excessive that some boys grow up to embody pathologically exaggerated ideas and attitudes about manhood. We reviewed the cycle of unmanageability, and how it can lead to greater isolation in the end. And we discussed the path of the hero, and how the ultimate goal of every man is to discover the hero that exists within.

Life for many men is a frustrating search for the part of themselves that has not learned what it feels like to be safe, nurtured, protected, and loved. The search can be all-consuming; it can crowd every thought with potent urgency. It can leave us distracted, aching for the position and the possessions of others. It creates a resistance to what the heart really wants.

But life does not have to be this way. We can begin a new narrative; we can start the conversation. Men cry. Men feel. Men grow. Our search for the man inside of each of us does not have to be distorted by our repressions, our compromises, our fears and our narcissistic manipulations.

Manhood 101

Men who want to scare the world into believing that masculinity is about power are struggling with feelings of weakness.

Men who do not know how to be soft and gentle with a woman are struggling with anger and hate.

Men who want to accumulate more and more with the aim that it will make them feel better are struggling with emptiness.

Men who fight, and control, and contend, and hurt one another are struggling with fear.

True masculinity is not about winning respect through force. It is about giving life to others, and creating relationships where love and intimacy are expressed without fear of rejection, shame, or abandonment. It is about honoring our parents for the sacrifices they made in raising us. It is about brotherhood and connection, mentoring and inspiration.

Manhood is ancestral; it contains voices of the past, credos and stories that beg for a re-instatement of the fallen world.

Manhood is spiritual; it contains a soul, which is the seat of our deepest emotions. It allows room for uncertainty, insecurity, and questioning while offering the opportunity for glory and redemption.

Manhood finds us hugging, dancing, and hoisting upon our shoulders the burdens of other people's sorrows.

It finds us crying and laughing. And it allows us to love with all our hearts, even the parts that still need repair.

Unworthiness and Fear

7

From childhood's hour I have not been

As others were—I have not seen

As others saw—I could not bring

My passions from a common spring—

From the same source I have not taken

My sorrow—I could not awaken

My heart to joy at the same tone—

And all I lov'd—I lov'd alone—

Edgar Allan Poe

E very one of us has a belief system that is fueled by assumptions about our world. Known in psychology as our **core beliefs**, these assumptions and suppositions are central to our identity. They consist of judgments, myths, personal truths, and even intergenerational messages, about our value and worth. They are the filter through which we make our decisions, interpret other people's actions, establish priorities, and behave in relationships. Our core beliefs range in depth from simple thoughts such as "life is hard" to complex cognitions about religion, spirit, and the meaning of our existence. They act as an "inner lawyer," superego, and moral compass, constantly affirming or disconfirming our feelings, behaviors, and choices.

But core beliefs can sometimes lead to cognitive distortions, or impaired thinking. Denial is a common example of an impaired thought process where we might minimize a behavior, ignore a problem, or justify an action erroneously.[49] These **defensive rationalizations** are often used in the service of protecting ourselves from deeper, more unacceptable feelings of shame or fear. They operate unconsciously, and, in the psyches of adults who were traumatized as children, occur because a healthy **internal feedback loop** has been silenced, shut off, or never fully developed. Thus, in an almost immediate sweep of unconscious surrender, we accept our faulty assumptions.

There is a cycle to our negative thoughts and faulty assumptions.[50] We may not be aware of the flow of ideas and subsequent actions as they are occurring, but the negative thoughts impact us nonetheless. Becoming more aware of this cycle can help all of us to begin the process of change. Below is a list of the unconscious interchange between mind and body:

Cycle of Negative Thinking

Early Trauma: Criticism, or other forms of negative attention, from a trusted adult or caretaker.

Automatic Belief: Unhelpful assumption or core belief about ourselves (e.g., "I am no good," "It is always my fault," or "I am unworthy").

Preoccupation: An unconscious trance or mood wherein we become engrossed with thoughts of unworthiness.

Ritualization: Routines that fortify or confirm our core belief (e.g., pursuing friends that will likely reject us).

Critical Incident Later in Life: Sudden or unexpected changes or stressors that alter our plan (e.g., relationship break-up; not getting the desired part in the play; being laid-off from work).

Negative Automatic Belief: Unconscious scripts that we repeat to ourselves silently (e.g., "It's all my fault," "This is how it always goes with me," "I'm a moron, a joke, a failure").

Despair: The feeling of utter hopelessness about our power to effect change.

Resulting Action: Social withdrawal, loss of motivation, little interest in everyday activities, anxiety, guilt, loss of appetite, negative self-soothing behaviors, and feelings of unworthiness resulting from a rejection or a failed attempt at something.

The pain we feel at the end of the cycle can be numbed or obscured by addictive actions such as alcohol consumption, drug use, sexual promiscuity, overeating, overspending, gambling, gaming, or other self-destructive behaviors.[51] This mode of self-soothing is ultimately met with disapproval (externally and/or internally), which only serves to reengage the early unconscious trauma—and the cycle begins again.

The Price of Unworthiness

Perhaps the most damaging automatic negative belief that survivors of abuse struggle with is a feeling of unworthiness. This feeling rises insidiously out of the unexpressed stories of the times when we were mistreated. As survivors, we are congested with these stories, and they generate fear, and even dread. They block access to our feelings of worth. As a result, we often find it hard to meet the demands of the day. We are humbled, and we feel low to the ground.

Immediately after the trauma occurred, many of us discovered that the world we used to live in no longer existed.[52] We learned to live in a new world without shape or reason. The person we knew ourselves to be was shockingly altered, and we walked with fear and uncertainty. Now, years later, after challenging the storms of adolescence and honoring the initiation rites of our adulthood, we still, at "off" moments, feel uncertain.

"Was he correct when he said no one will love me the way he did?" we ask ourselves of the abuser.

"Is it true that 'I asked for this,' or that I wanted it to happen?"

Even in the presence of rational adult thought, we still challenge our assumptions about ourselves. These thoughts, wrapped in shame, were banished to the deepest parts of our psyche.[53] And when they surface, we hate them. We refuse to allow them the light of day.

But when we deny their presence within us, we also deny the healing that can come from connection, truth, and healthy love. This is our predicament. We feel unworthy, but we are unable to share this feeling of unworthiness with anyone. And without a vital feedback system, such as a trusted parent, best friend, psychologist, or coach, our negative beliefs will likely repeat themselves, causing us to continue to feel outside the circle of worth.

Fact vs. Feeling

The key to our ability to change these feelings of unworthiness is to recognize them when they are happening. Then we challenge their veracity and ultimately release them from the grip they used to have on us.

1. Catch the negative statements as they occur. Most of us have unconscious scripts that we say to ourselves when events do not go the way we had planned (e.g., we discover that we were not invited to a friend's holiday party, and immediately we say to ourselves, "I am not good enough.").

Use the space below to write down an automatic negative belief that relates to a crisis in your life.

_____

_____

_____

_____

_____

_____

2. *Welcome the presence of this belief. This is a meditation practice that is designed to help you "outlast" the negative feeling.[54] When we attempt to push away our pain, we almost always find ourselves hurting more. The equation is: Pain + Resistance = Suffering. Therefore, this step asks that you stay with the feelings of discomfort for a while. Acknowledge them. Notice how they make you feel. What are they saying to you?*

_____

_____

_____

_____

_____

_____

3. *Know the science of your body. This current emotional state, and the corresponding negative feeling, was evoked by a threat that is likely filled with misinformation. When you are afraid, uncertain, or hurt, dopamine is being ignited in your brainstem. Now your mind and body are on high alert. Write down the physical symptoms you are experiencing in your body:*

_____

_____

_____

_____

_____

_____

4. Know the difference between a fact and a feeling. Feelings are organic arousal states to which assumptions are attributed. When dopamine is ignited, we are more prone to misinterpretation. We mis-attribute. Then, we assume the worst. Tell yourself: "This is only a feeling. It is *not* a fact. And therefore, I could be wrong."

5. Challenge that feeling. Repetition is the unspoken language of the abused child. This means that, as adults who were hurt in our youth, our biological instinct is to repeat what happened to us over and over. Thus, we are likely to repeat the same (mis) interpretation over and over. Recognize this. Acknowledge it. You are capable of being wrong about your interpretation. Remember: alternative interpretations *do* exist.

Exercises that involve meditation, imagery, and cognitive behavioral strategies help us to sort out the difference between a cascading flow of negative emotions from the facts as they *really* are. Known in Eastern spiritual practice as "wisely seeing," this exercise was designed to help you approach a situation from an impartial, nonjudgmental, fearless, and neutral point of view.

The desired outcome of the exercise was for you to be able to transform an emotionally disturbing belief into a *challenge*. This can be immensely therapeutic. The estranged, or repressed, parts of your shameful memories have been filtered out, and now you can strategize a healthy plan with a wiser mind.

Mahatma Gandhi once said,

I do not want to see the future. I am concerned with taking care of the present. God has given me no control over the moment following.

Finding peace in the midst of a stressful moment or day is not about adding another task to our already too-long to-do list. It is a choice, and a gift, that we give to ourselves. We choose to be alert, to bring our attention to this moment *only*.

Breathe. And allow this moment to be a peaceful one. In this way, you will declutter your mind and rise above your fixed, erroneous views.

. . . .

The next part of the chapter is devoted to understanding a related symptom of trauma, namely fear. Fear, in all of its manifestations, is the touchstone of trauma—in the advancement of its impact on the victim, and also in its origin. Devastating mistreatment in childhood is the genesis of the fear we feel as adult survivors, and it has damaging effects on our daily functioning.

One common phenomenon of fear is known as the fight-or-flight response, which is the body's automatic reaction to an actual or perceived threat of danger (most often life-threatening). This frightening event overwhelms our personal theory of the world, and it compromises our normal or usual coping abilities. Physiologically, our sympathetic nervous system is being activated, causing us to either fight the danger or to flee for safety.[55] In addition, the language center in our brain (Broca's area) shuts down. We become literally struck "dumb," or mute with fear. Additionally, our memory center (hippocampus) fills up with cortisol, thus rendering us less able to remember the events as they happen.

A second side effect of fear is that self-reliance and independent thinking quickly evaporate; we question our choices, decisions, and intentions. We hear the faint voices from our past calling out our foibles and reminding us of our missteps. We thus begin to question our power and competence. We are more vulnerable to releasing our power to those who appear more charismatic and confident.[56]

A third observable occurrence is a sense of being accompanied by a second self—a critical observer who lives alongside of us but does not share the insecurities that we have. He walks with dispassionate curiosity as we struggle to keep our demons inside.[57] This person always knows the right thing to say, or has the confidence to speak up when we do not; and we wish we could be more like this fantasy-self.

A fourth phenomenon of fear is our intense need for acceptance and support. Like a hunter in search of prey, our hungry soul seeks validation and consolation for unmet needs from our youth. But the hunt is not easy, for we are bound to be met by unwelcome memories and forbidden feelings that were neatly, carefully, buried inside of the past.

These fears, remnants of a childhood where bad things happened, stand in the path of restored serenity and peace. We tell ourselves that we will succeed in ways that are different from our childhood. We look for reasons to be happy, and we pray for things to work out for us in the end. But all too often, old familiar feelings of fear pop up like jack-in-the-boxes, threatening to challenge our goals for a happy life.[58]

The following is a list of the more common fears that survivors of child abuse find themselves struggling with. Each description is followed by an exercise that is designed to help you to explore ways to manage these fears more effectively.

Fear of Intimacy

Attempts at intimacy pose a great threat to those of us who have been abused as children, for it is in the context of intense emotional attachments that our darker secrets suddenly reappear. This is because the closer we come to another person, the closer we come to our own inner selves. And this internal movement forces old patterns and conflicts to resurface, threatening to challenge the peace we thought we had found.

It is at these times that we dig in our heels and argue incessantly, or we run away from our partner (fight, flight, or freeze). Unbeknownst to us, we are being triggered. Feelings that we tucked away are now strangely revisiting us, and we are reactivated and afraid. Sometimes we even see in our mate eerie resemblances of the abuser, or of someone whom we knew and feared in the past.

Simply stated, our partner sometimes serves as a mirror of ourselves. When we are unhappy with ourselves, we believe our partner feels this way about us, too. Thus, we feel compelled to manipulate the mirror through fighting, in order to bring about a more tolerable, if only momentary, view of ourselves.

Climbing the Ladder

In trauma therapy, this exercise is akin to climbing six rungs of a ladder:

1. Retrace your childhood steps (and missteps) and acknowledge the things that were done to you, and not *by* you. Tell your younger self, "It wasn't your fault." The baggage you carry (negative beliefs and thoughts about self) were forced upon you by a person who was forced to carry them from someone else in *his or her* life. Remember: Fear is an STD—a **S**elfish **T**ransmission of **D**isgrace.

2. Repair the survival instinct that you were born with. This is the voice inside of you that assures you that you are capable, and worthy, and just. This is the instinct that was injured from those who hurt you when we were young and unknowing.

3. Nurture new lessons about life, particularly the lesson of revenge. Revenge is an evil spirit that keeps the path open toward unending animus and rage. Evil does not go away when you "get even." The need for vengeance makes you hateful. When you seek retribution through anger, you absent yourself from good.[59]

4. Speak up for what you believe in, for the values and ethics that you stand for. Seek out peers, fellow survivors, who have similar fears to yours. Support groups have been established and designed for those who once lived in darkness. Some are quite helpful, for they offer a chance to speak a common language with others who truly understand.

5. Bear being misunderstood, for you are learning and growing every day. Remember, you are worthy and deserving of *healthy love*. Look upon those who judge you as needing your mercy, and your prayers. Your partner's erroneous views of you are likely borne of his or her own inner fears.

6. Be confident in your interchanges. You may appear mild and demure on the outside, but you are really boundless in your ideas, dreams, and desires deep within. Reclaim what was taken from you; your inner sight, your instinctual drive to heal and grow, and your natural force to succeed in this life you were gifted.

Thus, in embracing your fear of intimacy, you recognize that beneath all things, no matter how awful, goodness *does* exist. Look upon yourself with compassion, tolerance, and understanding. Challenge the actions of those who counter you, but do so in ways that help them turn their own darkness into a light for the world. And when you do these things with integrity and with a full heart, you ready yourself for intimacy with someone you love. For the full spectrum of light exists in the union of two healthy souls.

Fear of Betrayal

Many of us idealize a partner, a lover, or someone we are dating. We tell ourselves that we finally found the love we have been searching for our whole lives. We run quickly into a relationship with this person, and for a while, a "honeymoon phase," we experience the joy and validation that comes from new love.

But sometimes people disappoint. The hope we had of this relationship "saving" us from our inner demons becomes questionable, for our partner is also human, and they have their own inner fears and unexamined needs to conquer. Eventually, the feeling of betrayal sets in. As the relationship waxes and wanes, we discover that we may have been seeking out a love object who was different from the person we had originally believed they were.

"It will be different this time," we tell ourselves.

"Love will save me," we pray.

This "theft of the heart" causes us to think that we are at fault.[60] But this may be the furthest thing from the truth. We who have been hurt are not bad people, and we have not done anything to deserve this negative treatment. Our only role in this rejection process may have come from being overly optimistic, having had unrealistic expectations of our partner, or having been lost in some kind of "psychic slumber." We can blame ourselves for being naive, or for not noticing the signs along the way. But this "theft" was not our fault, and it is not our guilt to carry.

Self-Forgiveness

The key to healing our fear of betrayal is to locate our inner power and forgive ourselves for the mistakes of others. However, there are two obstacles that impede our ability to forgive ourselves:

1. The first is our belief that self-forgiveness means that we are letting ourselves "off the hook." Specifically, many of us think that, the more critical and judgmental we are of ourselves, the more inspired we will be to change or improve. But this is the opposite of the truth, for the more self-critical we are, the more self-loathing we become; hence, the *less* we will improve.

Therefore, **let yourself off the hook**. Growing up scared created a spiral of negative beliefs that brought you down. You felt inept, incapable, hopeless, and unworthy. The voices in your head told you that you were bad. While none of this was true, it affected you deeply. Now is the time to allow yourself to silence the critic.

What statements were you made to believe about yourself that were never true to begin with?

_____

_____

_____

_____

_____

_____

Now that you have listed these statements, recognize that they are not emanating from you. They are words that were spoken *to* you, or *around* you, by someone who was filled with his or her own self-hate. Rewrite these statements. This time, imagine that you are returning these statements back to the person(s) who wrongly said them to you. This is the origin of your self-hate. Return these words as if they were an unclaimed Amazon package left by mistake on your doorstep.

The statements are to be rewritten in a new form. "I am" statements are now transformed into "You are" statements. Imagine you are saying good-bye to these erroneous beliefs. You are returning them to their original owner.

_____

_____

_____

_____

_____

2. The second obstacle to healing our fear of betrayal is our belief that we need to be perfect. Growing up either witnessing or experiencing abuse resulted in our belief

that "being perfect" would keep us safe. But this is not true, for we are all human and are, therefore, all gloriously imperfect. We go from strength to weakness, and from weakness to strength.

Life presents itself to us in a variety of colors, including all shades of gray. And as we grow, we are being asked to resist the temptation to divide our world into black and white, or good and bad, or perfect and imperfect.

Write down aspects of yourself that are flawed. Write them down with pride, for, as the Persian poet Rumi once said, "The cracks are where the light comes through."

_____

_____

_____

_____

_____

Fear of Engulfment

Many of us want to help a friend in need. But as we listen and attempt to hold their pain for them, we absorb their energy, as well as the words that they are saying. As a result, our compassion leaves us feeling tired, spent, or even overwhelmed. What we do not realize is that we are becoming imprinted with the negative energy that they are emanating; this information can move us, and impact us, in bad ways.

Suddenly, an unconscious shift occurs in our identity. Our original wish to help our partner causes us to lose a sense of ourselves as *separate* from our mate. The result is a momentary fusion with them; we "lose ourselves" in a sea of their sorrow. We fear that we will be swallowed up and disappear.

Our natural reaction to this fear is to run. We become distant, we shut down. The withdrawal happens automatically and unconsciously, until a new difficulty develops: we begin to feel empty and alone. Thus, we swing back. We move *closer* to our partner, and the swing of the pendulum repeats itself indefinitely.

This is a dialectic that is as old as history itself. Perhaps the first example of this "approach-avoidant" attachment style is in the Bible, where Jonah, who ran from God, was engulfed by a whale. While inside the belly of that deep unknown, Jonah cried out, claiming that he would rather die than suffer a life of darkness.

But darkness carries within it the seeds of possibility, and of undiscovered wisdom and truth. Like Jonah, love asks us to *fall* into the belly of the unknown. But this is scary for many of us. We may not feel ready to connect with others. In order to be able to tolerate closeness with others, we must first become more mindfully self-aware.

Mindful Self-Awareness

As we said in the beginning of this chapter, our struggles in life depend a great deal on our core beliefs and values. Some core values are relational, such as honesty, generosity, and service to others. Other core values are personal, such as spiritual growth, integrity, and musical expression. This exercise is designed to help you remember what your core values are, and whether you are living in sync with them. When we live in alignment with our core values, we find that we are less susceptible to fears of engulfment (being inexorably pulled by the needs and wants of others to the point of losing ourselves).

Imagine that you are in your elder years and you are reviewing all you have achieved. Perhaps you are sharing with a grandchild, or other young person, all the important things you learned about yourself in life. Looking back, you feel a deep sense of satisfaction at these things. You recognize and praise yourself for the obstacles you overcame, and you honor those moments when you stayed true to yourself.

Use the space below to write down the core values you have learned through life:

Reflection: Notice how this exercise made you feel. You may have struggled to identify some of your core values and beliefs. You may have noticed that some core values were not truly your own but, rather, values that others told you you *should* have. You may still need to discover what you truly stand for and what you believe in. In addition, you may need to separate your *own* personal beliefs from those of others who may have been overly persuasive in your youth. This reflection will help you manage fears of getting "too close" to others, for among all other things, you must always know *who you are*, and what *you stand for*.

Fear of Abandonment

Anxiety over separation is a built-in, instinctual mechanism in all human beings.[61] Sociobiologically, this mechanism kept us, as a species, from wandering away from the pack, and out of danger. Thus, we have an instinctual need for union, togetherness, and belonging.

In healthy child development, this need for union is accomplished through safe and appropriate interactions with our caretaker. The caretaker, our first real love object, becomes an orienting figure; our mother and/or father become our home base in the world.

But when this attachment is ruptured (through trauma, abuse, illness, death, or divorce), our dream of paradise is lost. The feelings of security and safety that usually blossom in the union between parent and child are ruined, and we begin to develop an expectation that *love is not always safe.*

This becomes our automatic belief as we grow into adulthood. We tell ourselves that we "will be found out," and we thus become hypervigilant to the threat of being left alone. All of this is occurring in our frightened mind, which is filled with the fears of insecurity and self-defeat. The rupture we experienced in our early attachment years (likely created by someone who defined or "branded us" as "bad, dispensable, and unlovable") has us believing that will be abandoned again and again. We cannot regulate our feelings effectively, and a fight ensues in which old intimacies—shards of intensely emotional hurts from our childhood—reemerge and destroy the peace we so badly wanted to experience. The paradox here is that the closeness we crave becomes the very reason we may run away, and a resolution will never be reached.

Challenging the Sword

According to the legend of Cicero, a glittering sword was suspended above the head of a young man named Damocles, who wanted to experience the rich and powerful lifestyle of the king. At the king's behest, Damocles was granted the right to sit upon his throne, but with one condition: A sword was to be hung in midair above Damocles, held at the handle by the single hair of a horse's tail. Young Damocles accepted the offer.

But as time ensued, he could think about nothing else but the specter of tragedy that would befall him if the thin horsehair were to suddenly snap. Damocles eventually became disenchanted with his place on the throne, as his only thought turned to whether he would be annihilated, left for dead, or worse, left unloved and unsafe.

This story exemplifies how some of us feel when we fear our loved one will abandon us. We consider it a fate worse than death. This happens because we are lacking strong principles of self-worth and self-love. Thus, the exercise below is designed to help you reinstate your once-fallen power.

Use the space below to list these personal strengths and virtues. Answer the question: "Who am I when I am at my very best?

As you write down each "personal best" strength, imagine each statement as an invincible cord of steel that will be used to fasten the sword of Damocles to its handle. Your own list of worthiness will act as the tether that yokes the sword to its base. This meditation offers you a method of reigniting your personal virtues while strengthening your ability to self-soothe. Together, these are the qualities that will bring you closer to relief from fear.

_____

_____

_____

_____

_____

_____

Remember: You are worthy. You are stronger than you know. And you are loved.

In this chapter we have reviewed the origin, as well as the symptoms of our feelings of unworthiness and fear. We discussed the cycle of negative thinking, and the price we all pay when we allow our automatic negative thoughts to take over our "wise mind." We worked on exercises to help us distinguish the facts from the feelings, as well as to discern effective ways to climb the ladder of self-love, confidence, and power. Fear has been our unbidden companion through time. It is the orphan child of trauma and abuse, but we know now that it no longer needs to stay by our side.

Some feelings and thoughts only emerge in darkness. Fear is one of them. Therefore, we naturally resist fear, for our reflections grow deeper in the dark, becoming distilled into a sense of who we *think* we are. We *think* we are monsters. We *think* we are unworthy. We *think* we are undeserving, even incapable, of healthy love.

But what if we redefined the meaning of fear? What if none of our primitive perceptions of fear were true? What if fear is really a *teacher*?

Faced with fear, we might ask it: "What are you doing here? Do you have some necessary role to play?"

Use the space below to answer these questions:

_____

_____

_____

_____

_____

_____

The answer to these very important questions will guide your way to recovery. For fear is *actually* an initiation, a rite of passage. As an alternative to our instinctual fight-or-flight response, we must consider inviting fear in when it comes knocking, to allow it access to our internal world without trying to change or interpret it.

When we sit with our fear for a while, when we meditate upon its core, we discover that it has a centrifugal force; it eventually moves away from the center—from *our* center. It is not a demon who came to redefine us as bad and unworthy. Rather, it is more like an angel who, unwelcomed and unashamed, came to help us grow.

The Childhood Trauma Recovery Workbook for Adults

Whether real, symbolic, spiritual, or imagined, we all struggle with the presence of a shadow—an energy that resounds from a place we cannot touch.[62] This is the Angel of Fear. And it summons us to act in ways that are, for better or worse, consistent with our soul's purpose. We are here to learn and to grow, and through our struggle we will one day achieve this noble goal.

Thus, we acknowledge our fear. We sit *with* it, we move forward *with* it, we evolve *with it*.

We breathe. We wait. And we watch as it weaves its lessons into our developing, growing sense of self. We are learning that we are good people, pure in our deepest core.

When we fear, we take a breath, and we tell ourselves, "I am about to learn something."

This is worthiness.

8

Addiction and Self-Harm

Why I ingested chemical waste? It was a kind of desire to abbreviate myself...I wanted to be less, so I took more— simple as that.

Carrie Fisher, *Wishful Drinking* (2008)

One of the greatest casualties of surviving a trauma in childhood is that our brain develops an involuntary need for a reward system that clouds our awareness of any and all feelings and thoughts that can hurt us.[63] This reward system becomes automatic and repetitive, especially if it has inherent pleasurable consequences. Understood in this way, an addiction is a habitual response, and a source of gratification and security. It is our way of coping with internal feelings and external pressures.

The driving thought of the addict is *"I gotta have it!"*[64] Whether it is a drink, a drag, a hit, a line, or a piece of chocolate, a **craving response** is set in place. **Craving** is an uncomfortable, obsessional reaction to an event that compels us to act out so we can attain a desired outcome. Neurologically, our primitive survival system sends a message to the brain, telling it that things are out of balance. The message comes in the form of a dopamine release, which puts the body in **action mode**. It is a battle for survival. Under ordinary circumstances, this "battle" protects us from danger or distress. It forces us to engage in efficient, goal-directed behavior. But this battle also comes from moments of emotional distress and ego confusion. When this happens, we become stuck in **search mode**.[65] The greater the stress, the greater the brain's search for satisfaction and relief.

Addictive behaviors include the following four elements:

- They represent habitual and compulsive patterns of intentional behavior.
- They ultimately produce negative consequences.
- There are interrelated psychological and physical components to the behavior.
- Stopping or modifying the behavior is highly difficult.

The addiction cycle flows in the following manner:

1. **The Trauma:** The abused child, now a teen, feels a lack of satisfaction in everyday life. He is deprived of family and community supports; he lacks self-confidence and has no compelling interests; and he struggles with feelings of depression and anxiety.

2. **The Draw:** Satisfying the craving response brings about feelings of gratification that cannot be achieved in other ways. Temporary relief, and feelings of calm and security, are the reward.

3. **The Cost:** The addict responds less and less to other people in his world. (The "real" world appears worse and worse to him.) As the addiction grows, he becomes more and more out of touch with the responsibilities of life.

4. **The Withdrawal:** When the addictive object is removed, the addict becomes deprived of his primary source of comfort. He may experience a "crash landing," which is characterized by self-loathing and self-blame.

5. **The Credo:** He begins to believe that the addiction is stronger than he is. He can find no other meaningful alternatives. Hopelessness about the future sets in.

This introduction to the definition, and the etiology, of addiction is the foundation of your ability to work through this current chapter. Gaining a better understanding of how your addiction impacted your life can help you to change the belief, or credo, that you held onto in the past or that you may still be holding onto at this moment. Thus, we ask you to answer the following questions:

What is the addiction you are/were involved in? How did it make you feel?

_____

_____

_____

_____

_____

In the space below, describe how the cycle of addiction played out for you:

The Trauma:

_____

_____

_____

The Draw:

_____

_____

_____

The Cost:

_____

_____

_____

The Withdrawal:

_____

_____

_____

The Credo:

_____

_____

_____

Substance Abuse

Drugs and alcohol make up the most common form of addiction. Research on addiction in our culture reveals that drug use most often begins as an innocent act of rebellion or social initiation.[66] Children are offered a beer or are handed a joint and all involved assume it is part of the rite of passage into adolescence and adulthood. Many children and teens who are introduced to alcohol and drugs continue to use them occasionally, while others use them frequently. Some become addicted.

These are the numbers:[67]

- More than twenty million people in America are addicted to drugs.
- Approximately one in twelve Americans over age twelve is addicted to drugs.
- Everyday drugs kill over 365 Americans.
- Drugs are linked to more ER visits than any other single hospital visit.
- In 2010, 85 percent of US prisons were filled with criminals who committed crimes while under the influence of alcohol or drugs.
- Drugs are involved in over 50 percent of child abuse and domestic violence crimes.

All stages of the lifecycle have their unique and particular stressors, and adolescence is an exceptionally difficult one. When abuse or trauma is introduced into a child's life, adolescence becomes fraught with unique internal pressures that mix with external temptations. The teen who was abused feels defeated, confused, alienated, and "different," and drugs become particularly appealing, as they offer a paradoxical promise. They help the teen find a way to live more comfortably in the "real" world, while they provide a numbing, less painful alternative world in which to hide.

Nicotine

According to *Never Enough: The Neuroscience and Experience of Addiction*, addiction may be the greatest health problem in America, affecting one in every five people of over the age of fourteen, and nicotine is often the first drug of choice.[68] The adapted brain makes it harder and harder to quit. In fact, cigarette smoking is harder to quit than other addictions. This is because it seems to fit more comfortably into ordinary lifestyle activities. Research reveals that the nicotine helps the addict to maintain balance under heightened levels of stress by "dampening" the emotional force of the pain he feels inside.

Unlearning the dependence to nicotine depends on the addict's appreciation of the dangers it poses to his health. Thus, education about heart and lung disease, and criticism by others about the aesthetic impact it has on his complexion, breath, and clothing, can help change his attitude about the addiction. The more decisive a smoker is about changing his attitude, the stronger becomes his ability to stop.

Food Addiction

Like addictive drugs, food can also trigger changes in the release of dopamine in the brain. Specifically, once the addict experiences pleasure from a certain food, the brain's reward pathway signals pleasure sensations that override our feelings of fullness and satisfaction. The result is that we eat more, only to discover that the food begins to satisfy us less. This activates a need to force the presence of the reward, and we eat to the point of feeling ill. We feel powerless over food, but we comfort ourselves with the knowledge that total abstinence from food is clearly impossible.

Emotional theories suggest that our physical image is linked to a statement about how we feel about ourselves.[69] Thus, when we are self-loathing, we are more prone to break our promise to maintain better nutrition. Our food addiction provides a predictable satisfaction for us when we feel "emotionally empty."

Love Addiction

Healthy love originates from healthy attachments between child and caretaker early in life. These primary connections provide a mechanism for us to regulate our emotions. Thus, if our caretaker was physically and emotionally available to us, we learned to feel loved. We told ourselves:[70]

"I know who I am, and I know where I belong."

These internal statements are important, for they are the foundation of mental health. They teach us to make meaning out of ambiguous moments between friends and lovers, and they help us to tolerate (live *through*) the discomfort of a fight or a bad feeling.

However, some of us were raised by a caretaker who was emotionally or physically unavailable. Others may have had a parent who was inconsistent in his or her ability to meet our primitive needs. Thus, we grew up craving external validation for our self-worth and, now, as adults, we find ourselves saying to our partner:

"Tell me you love me."

"Promise me that you won't leave me."

This type of needfulness will hurt the relationship, for it creates an imbalance of power in the pair. The unregulated partner will languish on the emotional level of a "child" whose needs are too great for the "adult" partner to meet. What ultimately develops are feelings of exhaustion, disenchantment, and a detachment from one another.

It is important that we do not turn to our lover or partner to numb us from our internal pain. Instead, we must learn to turn inward and self-sooth, to make meaning out of ambiguous moments in the relationship. Breathe. Tolerate feelings of uncertainty and develop ways to be a clearer thinker.

Take care of yourself before you ask your partner to take care of you.

Sexual Addiction

Sex addiction is parallel to alcoholism and drug dependency in that the addict uses—or abuses—sexual arousal in order to alter his mood. Metabolic changes create a rush through the body as the addict focuses on his search for the "object." This is known as euphoric recall, and it refers to the positive sensation the addict receives when he simply thinks about his plan.[71] The "excitement-seeking" thoughts and actions are triggered through the fantasy, as well as the pursuit, and the conquest.

Eventually, as with all addictions, the sex addict discovers that he is powerless over his needs. This recognition adds to his inner shame, and despair sets in. There is a feeling of failure, a letdown over not being able to stop this behavior (which sometimes includes degrading, humiliating, or risky sexual activity). Self-hatred sets in, and the need to numb this feeling restimulates the cycle all over again.

Compulsive cybersex or porn addiction is part of the arousal cycle as well. Hence, the keyboard or the cellphone, or our favorite website, become associated with the adrenal changes in our body. Porn abuse creates distortions in our neuropathways; we can become aroused in ways that are destructive, unrealistic, and un-translatable to real life.[72] Moreover, our neurons go on overload, for we are filling our brains with more information that it was designed to handle. Depression, loneliness, and despair eventually meet us at the end of our obsessional marathon, and we realize we are trapped in a cycle that has to stop.

Addiction in the Couple

Addictive behaviors pay a heavy toll on the couple, and the addict's denial of the problem will become a problem for the pair. Denial is a defense mechanism that justifies the addict's continued use of his or her vice. Cognitive impairments, impulsive actions, and enabling behaviors between the partners all become part of the problem.

This generally culminates in an unconscious collusion between the addict and the partner—a dangerous dance which has consequences. This is because, in an effort to maintain peace in the home, the non-addict will likely respond benevolently to the "devil" that the addict has inside. This will, in turn, awaken the devil inside of the "overhelping" mate. Known by psychologists and couples' therapists as **pathological nurturance**, this dance allows the addicted partner to manipulate the other in the name of their own unconscious survival needs:[73]

> "I will continue to look away from your addiction," cries the mate unconsciously, "If you continue to allow me to act on my addictions."

This dance is happening usually out of the couple's awareness. It is thus imperative at these times that each member of the pair embrace their role in the collusion. They must say to each other:

> "My shit is back and I have work to do to get healthy."

Couples who honor the presence of their addictions, and speak openly about the emotions and experiences that are kicked up as a result of them, will get healthier as they each find ways to get clean.

Prepare for Change

Change is possible. Healing does happen. It occurs in stages and it involves commitment and discipline.

1. Planning: This stage of change involves decision making. We must develop a plan of action that is reasonable and feasible to execute. It involves self-observation, and monitoring our feelings and our impulsive responses. We must begin to avoid places and people associated with our addictive behaviors. In addition, we create a list of the changes we wish to make and why:

The changes I want to make are:

_____

_____

_____

_____

The most important reasons for making these changes are:

_____

_____

_____

_____

2. Include others: This stage involves searching for alternative reinforcers when stress arises, such as trusted family members, religious affiliations, or work-related activities that support our desire to change. Connection with others ensures that we will not fall again. This is a necessary part of our recovery.

The people I choose to help me are:

_____

_____

_____

_____

The ways these people can help me are:

_____

_____

_____

_____

3. Define the characteristics of change: The goal of this stage is to establish new patterns of behavior. Some markers of change in our recovery from addiction include feelings of self-effectiveness. This involves measuring the confidence we feel in our ability to stop the addiction. It also includes feelings of power or control that we have in other areas of life.

Write down the changes you feel you are already making in this process (e.g., self-effectiveness, increased confidence, meeting new friends, staying away from old connections that were bad for me).

_____

_____

_____

_____

4. Take Action: The important task at this stage is to break away from the addictive behavior and to create new ways of relating. Action begins now. Leaving an addiction feels a lot like leaving an intense love relationship. The feelings of familiarity and security are being severed. It takes time and energy to sever these connections, and romancing the old addiction will be temping. We must not allow ourselves to renew ties with the old addiction.

Write down what actions you will take when nostalgia for the old addiction creeps into your mind. Who can you call? What can you do to regain your sense of power and confidence over the old behaviors?

_____

_____

_____

_____

_____

This exercise was designed to help you start on the road to a cleaner, healthier life. It is intended as a beginning guide only. But there are many ways you can recover from addiction.

Some researchers in the field of addiction suggest that the first action to take is to enter an inpatient program to protect yourself from physiological dangers associated with recovery. Numerous detox programs and rehabilitation centers exist, and they are quite effective in helping addicts regain control over their lives. Contact your physician, psychologist, or clergy for help in finding an inpatient program that may be right for you.

Another perspective for recovery from addiction is promoted in the materials describing the twelve steps and twelve traditions of Alcoholics Anonymous (AA). The steps are individual instructions for recovery; each contains the goals of finding peace with ourselves, with God, and with others around us. As we climb these symbolic steps, we recognize our brokenness, we develop greater faith in a higher power, and we use self-examination to help us make amends for wrongdoings that hurt others. These steps invoke an ability for transformation and purification of our character and our actions. It is a program that helps addicts deepen the spiritual parts of themselves. The goal is to maintain freedom from addiction by learning to live your life according to the guidance of a higher power. AA support groups have helped countless people to overcome addiction and regain balance and improved health in their lives.

Are you currently in some form of therapy, rehabilitation program, or mindfulness technique center?

_____

_____

What changes have come from these programs?

_____

_____

_____

_____

_____

Do you have a good community of people (family or group members) around you?

_____

_____

If the answer was yes, what support do they give, and how do they make you feel?

_____

_____

_____

_____

_____

The Childhood Trauma Recovery Workbook for Adults

If the answer was no, what will it take for you to get into a program? Are you ready to take the leap?

_____

_____

_____

_____

_____

Understand that addicts are not bad people. For far too long, those of us with addictions have been judged as selfish and bad. This is simply untrue. We are good people who are struggling with a chronic and progressive disease. It is important that we do not blame ourselves, but rather, seek out the help that is available to end the cycle of destruction. Go to a doctor who is trained in addiction medicine. Choose evidence-based treatments such as those found in inpatient detox and rehabilitation programs. Or try AA, and remember that connection to a higher power and a spiritual process has helped countless people to overcome their addictions.

There are internal and external factors that drive us to use substances, food, gambling, shopping, sex, and love as a means for eradicating our pain. The most important prevention strategy is knowledge. We must all go forward with greater information and learned wisdom. This part of our chapter was created to help you gain access to some of that wisdom. With knowledge comes power. With power comes the ability to say no.

The great F. Scott Fitzgerald once wrote:

> *Tomorrow we will run faster, arms stretched out farther, and so we beat on, like boats against the current, born ceaselessly into the past.*

We all stand on the edge of life and valiantly face what lies ahead. We follow in the footsteps of our parents, our teachers, and our heroes while we struggle to find our own path. Our wish is to start anew, to discover a place that is wholly ours, different and untrammeled. And with wisdom, hard work, and a belief in a higher self or a higher power, we will find that new and untrammeled place. And we will call that place our "healthy connection."

. . . .

The next part of this chapter is devoted to understanding a related symptom of addiction, namely self-harm. Psychiatrist, trauma researcher, and author Bessel van der Kolk, MD, asserts that children who have a history of sexual and physical abuse are more prone to self-injurious behaviors, such as cutting, skin picking, and binge eating, as well as suicidal ideations. The most common predictor of whether a child will grow to develop self-destructive behaviors, he says, is having little to no memory of feeling safe in the presence of a caretaker. Having been frequently ignored or abandoned, molested, or beaten leave scars of unworthiness and a sense of defectiveness.[74] Thus, if we lack a deep memory of feeling loved and protected in our childhood, the receptors in our brain that react to human kindness simply fail to develop. The result is an inability to self-soothe or to create moments of internal peace.

—————————————————— EXERCISE 20 ——————————————————

Learning to Remember

Initiation leads to intimidation, which leads to isolation and mis-remembering. This is the path upon which survivors of child abuse travel. Attempts at sharing the terrible secret of what happened to them (or is still happening) may be met by adults who do not believe, or who consider it an exaggeration. Disruptions in memory eventually develop, and the hurt child will find himself saying such statements as "That didn't happen to me."

Disorders of memory are a child's way of helping him avoid or survive the pain he feels.[75] Neurologically, the brain fills up with cortisol during abuse or threat of danger, thereby reducing the size of the hippocampus (the memory center) by 12 percent.[76] The result is a wavering certainty of how the traumatic events actually unfolded. Left without validation and support, the child withdraws more and more from a world that will not let him remember.

The following exercise is designed to provide you with internal validation for memories of a time when you were hurt but no one believed you. It is also designed to help you find, deep within the hidden past, one or two memories of human kindness (or a recollection of a safe adult who may have shown you care and concern), for these are the memories that will help you heal.

Remember: Trauma is not stored in the brain as a story with a beginning, a middle, and an end. Flashbacks are more likely the way we remember a trauma. These are isolated fragments of the experience that appear out of context. In the space below, write down momentary memories of your story if you feel safe enough to remember.

_____

_____

_____

_____

_____

In the space below, now write down the one or two (or more) memories you have of someone who acted toward you with human kindness. Developing awareness and cultivating episodes of kindness in your youth are healthy ways to gain a sense of trust and faith in the world. If you cannot remember a person or a time when you felt safe, think about a friend or therapist who in the present day has shown you healthy love and kindness. What did/do they say to you? How did/do they make you feel?

_____

_____

_____

_____

_____

You may notice that some of the words and images you wrote created a sense of discomfort inside of you. This is because your brain is trying to find a way to express what was once unspeakable. Take a moment to rest, as the re-exposure to some of these memories can be frightening and disorganizing. This is a good time to regain a sense of calmness.

Breathe. Pay attention to the muscles in your body. If you are feeling any tension at this moment, let it go by breathing it away. You are safe. Allow the developing feeling of safety to spread throughout your body. Remember, you are reading this workbook because you have a strong will, and ability, to heal. Tell yourself that you are worthy and loved.

. . . .

Understanding the Science Behind Self-Harm

We all contain a chemical storehouse in our brains. One group of chemicals, known as endogenous opioids, ignites during moments of intense fear and trauma. Thus, when we experience an abuse in childhood, opioids begin to surge inside of us and create a post-traumatic stress response (fight, flight, or freeze). As we grow further away from that trauma, the opioid system diminishes in our brain, and we go through a withdrawal, not unlike drug withdrawal.

But in our adulthood, we may be triggered by moments of fear or the threat of danger. At these moments, there is an acceleration of the opioid system once again in our brain, and we find ourselves gradually becoming addicted to the charge we receive by the negative event. While we know the negative charge is bad for us, our brain is telling us that it is familiar and even strangely stimulating.

Self-harm thus becomes a powerful, albeit negative, self-soothing mechanism. By hurting ourselves, we are creating alterations in our autonomic arousal system.[77] Thus, we binge and then purge; we cut or pick at our skin; or we go through episodes of reckless drug and alcohol abuse, or engage in compulsive and risky sexual behaviors. This is the mind and body's way of managing, or regulating, these out-of-control, primitive, and frightening emotions. Simply stated, through self-injury, we are attempting to re-create the endogenous opiate charge we once received as a child by creating a jolt to our nervous system. The familiar feeling comes over us as relief but is only temporary. We eventually come to discover that the emotional comfort we seek through this manner cannot be fully achieved.

Research has shown how victims of abuse often feel disconnected from their bodies. The neuroimaging studies of Dr. Bessel van der Kolk, for example, have revealed that trauma early in life causes the brain to shut down areas that transmit visceral feelings of pain. Specifically, in our effort to hide from terrifying effects of the abuse, we learned to deaden our ability to feel. Thus, self-harm becomes a desperate, albeit maladaptive, attempt to "feel again."[78]

What modes of self-harm have you found yourself employing to overcome your pain?

_____

_____

_____

_____

_____

How did these efforts make you feel?

_____

_____

_____

_____

_____

Write down a list of alternatives (safe methods of behavior that you can employ when you feel a need for autonomic arousal, such as going for a run, getting in touch with the elements of nature, or going for a bike ride):

_____

_____

_____

_____

_____

Emotions vs. Actions

As we have clarified above, emotions are chemical signals in our body that alert us to what is happening inside and around us. They carry neurological impulses that create an urge to act. Simply stated, when we are scared, we feel compelled to overcome the threat. Sometimes this threat actually requires an action, and sometimes it does not. This exercise is designed to help you discern the level of threat, and whether or not it demands an action.

It is our human tendency to believe that strong emotions are confirming a truth about a situation. This is called **emotional reasoning**,[79] and it reflects an erroneous assumption that a heightened arousal state is equal to a heightened threat of danger. But this is not always true. In fact, anxiety makes liars out of many of us. When we are stressed, our brains fill with neurotransmitters that are capable of confusing our clarity of thought. Oftentimes, there is no relationship between the strength of an emotion and any real threat or danger.

On the left-hand side of the space below, write down an emotion that generated extreme fear or distress in you. Give the intensity of this emotion a "threat-score" on a scale of 1 to 10. Then, on the right-hand side, write down whether that threat ever came to fruition.

EMOTION AND THREAT-SCORE	HOW IT TURNED OUT IN THE END

When we force ourselves to notice our feelings without judging them, we come to discover that they have less power over us. We are slowing down the emotional process by naming the feeling, quantifying its power, and then examining the actual outcome—and whether our actions were ever really merited. Focusing on the outcome of a situation can help us to curb our impulsive need to act.

This is known in cognitive behavioral therapy as **self-talk**.[80] We speak to ourselves and assess the reality of our fears. We remember how the situation turned out in the past. We assess how we felt about having performed an action related to our fear. And in the end, we become more capable of making healthier decisions.

Remember: Facts are not feelings. We never act on feelings. We only act on fact.

In this chapter we have reviewed the effect that child abuse has on the developing brain of the survivor. We learned how the neurotransmitters are engaged during traumatic moments, which give rise to an involuntary need for a reward system that serves to numb the pain. In addition, we discussed the emotional and psychological events that occur to create a cycle of craving.

The addictions vary depending upon the person and the environment, but in the aggregate, we see how addictive behaviors pay a heavy toll on individuals, couples, and families. Methods of recovery, including cognitive efforts that involve planning for necessary changes, and then taking action, will help us begin to break away from the addictive cycle. When we discover that we cannot do this effectively on our own, we consider alternative methods toward recovery, such as inpatient rehabilitation and/or a commitment to twelve-step programs that lean lovingly toward the support of a higher power.

All of these efforts involve connection to a community. Indeed, *the antidote to addiction is connection*. Think about it: the three most powerful words in the English language are "I hear you." Thus, when we become brave enough to surrender our old feelings of shame and insecurity to the heart and mind of a good friend, we become freed from our prison of loneliness and self-blame. We reach outward, and upward, and we *connect*. This teaches us that we are worthy, for our perceived brokenness is lovingly pieced together by the sacred ears of a loving other.

This is community.

Education

9

Action without understanding only leads you back to darkness.

B. Bryan Post

Research on trauma in childhood has produced a significant amount of empirical information regarding the development, impact, and treatment of child abuse for survivors and their families. The field of study is still ongoing, as psychologists, educators, physicians, and mental health counselors continue to bring forth new and promising clinical and theoretical insights. These insights reflect the views of a diverse group of thinkers and writers and, while some differences in conceptualization do exist, there are a number of absolute findings that unite this work. This is what is known as the clinical, or **empirical data**.

A second form of education comes from **lived experience**. This is insight that is gained through practice in the field, as well as through the sharing of stories of abuse and recovery, and the wisdom that is to be found there. The transmission of lessons learned through life experience is an essential part of emotional, intellectual, and spiritual growth. We must continue to educate ourselves and others, as these lessons will embed themselves into the depths of the listeners, and they will be continually taught to future generations.

Lessons learned from Empirical Data

Definitions of child abuse must acknowledge that it is an event of maltreatment, or a failure to act against maltreatment, carried out by an adult who abuses his power and trust. The definitions must include that the abuse is conducted, without consent or assent, on dependent, developmentally immature children and adolescents in violent ways that are indefensible.

Each state in the US is responsible for providing its own definitions of child abuse and neglect. In the aggregate, most states recognize four major types of maltreatment:

1. Physical abuse

2. Sexual abuse

3. Emotional abuse

4. Neglect

Many states identify the following variables in their definition as well:

5. Abandonment

6. Parental substance use

7. Human trafficking

Perpetrators of abuse include family members, professionals with whom a child has contact (e.g., teachers, coaches, youth group leaders), or other adults who may connect with children (e.g., babysitters or shopkeepers). The abuse can manifest in many ways, occur almost anywhere, and involve myriad inappropriate actions.

All states require that professionals, including teachers, physicians, social workers, mental health-care workers, childhood providers, and law enforcement officers act as mandatory reporters. The circumstances under which mandatory reporters are required to make the report vary between states, but all states concur that a report must be made when there is a reason to believe abuse has taken place.

The Centers for Disease Control and Prevention offers a list of risk factors for victimization and perpetration by caretakers. Below is a small but important compendium of these factors. Specifically, caregivers, and other adults who are at great risk for mistreating a child struggle with many of the following concerns:

1. Drug and alcohol abuse

2. Mental health difficulties, including depression and thought disorder

3. Poor understanding of a child's developmental needs

4. Were abused or neglected as children themselves

5. Low education and/or low income

6. Believe in using physical or corporal methods of discipline

7. Are isolated from extended family and/or friends

8. Live in unstable housing or have residents moving in and out frequently

The way a child will react to abuse will vary depending on the child's age; the length and extent of the actions; previous history of trauma or abuse; ; who the abuser was (was he/she known to the family or a stranger?); and how the disclosure of the abuse was handled. Many children will never tell anyone.

The above information is offered as empirically studied and peer reviewed data that is essential in our journey toward recovery, as well as prevention of future abuse. As stated above, lessons are also learned, and taught, through lived experiences, and we offer a section on this topic next.

Lessons from Lived Experience

Teaching the deeper, more personal lessons from our journey to healing invokes a sharing of our essence, our personal accomplishments, and the confidence we have gained in the process. Educating the world about child abuse and its damaging impact on all who are affected impels us into action. It forces us to reach out to others who may be hurting like we are. Through our efforts, we may even gain wisdom from our students, for spiritual and emotional knowledge does not flow in one direction only. Thus, when we educate others, we discover that we are not alone. We discover that there are many adults out there who walk a similar and parallel path, and they, too, are surviving.

Educating others about our lived experience has another powerful benefit in that it helps us to realize how much we have grown through the course of our suffering. This type of "outreach" will invariably restimulate moments of pain for us. This is because our exposure to the fears and struggles of others triggers within us memories of our darker days. But it can also help us to rediscover ourselves, and to reflect on how far we have come.

What are some of the important lessons (key points) that you have learned from this journey? You may wish to include lessons gleaned from journeying through this workbook as well. Consolidating our acquired wisdom and writing it down in one place is a powerful way of committing these lessons to memory. It also allows us to return to our writing when we need renewed support.

_____

_____

_____

_____

_____

_____

_____

_____

_____

_____

Wisdom gained through suffering and ultimate recovery is not ours to keep. It belongs to everyone. And as survivors of abuse, we know that we are merely guardians of the spiritual and emotional wisdom that was given—painfully—to us throughout this dark and important journey. Thus, when we are asked by survivors of abuse the age-old questions, "Why all of this suffering? What did I do to deserve this pain?" we offer a different kind of answer. We share our wisdom through kind moments of quiet compassion and timeless understanding. We sit in silence and we listen to their stories of sorrow, knowing all too well the journey that lies ahead of them.

Moreover, in our effort to educate the world, we discover that many of us, most of us, are on a common path. Teacher and student, master and disciple, we offer our light and emerge out of the darkness, both at the same time.

Use the space below to write down the wisdom that you gained as you emerged from your darkness:

_____

_____

_____

_____

_____

_____

_____

_____

_____

_____

"Not in Our Family"

We often hear of stories that are happening in other people's homes. This may include tragedies and traumas, divorce, drug abuse, child abuse, chronic illness, even death. And we say:

"This is not us. This type of thing doesn't happen in our family!"

But we are not necessarily correct when we say this. Our proclivity to deny these truths, our instinctual pull to say, "This is not us!" derives from an inability to tackle the threats and the dangers that come from self-awareness. Research reveals that in middle-class families, child abuse can often be covered up, not spoken about, or remain hidden in different ways. The "respectability" of such homes instills the credo that "these things do not happen in our house." In addition, families that are less likely to be known to the authorities or social work agencies generate less opportunity to be suspected of wrongdoing.[81]

There is no evidence that child abuse is confined to any one social class. However, abuse is more likely to occur in families that are chaotic (when a parent changes partners often, or where new relatives suddenly appear).[82]

Thus, we need to observe our family; we need to take a *closer* look and challenge the harmony that we believe is surrounding us. Perhaps some of us would stop from saying "This is not us" and instead say:

"This *could* be us...and we have work to do."

The Lessons Learned from "the Difficult Child"

As we continue to educate others about the impact of abuse, we must also recognize the effect the abuse has on the family system at large. Specifically, when child abuse occurs, the entire family is affected. The hurt child will act out and become unwittingly known as the "difficult one," or "the black sheep." He quickly becomes labeled as "different" from all the others. But this label, deserved or not, can have damaging effects on future functioning for all members of the group. And if we were the child who received this label, we will be at risk for classifying ourselves in this manner and, thus, fulfilling the prophecy in our future relationships.

A healthier way to understand the label of "the difficult child" is to see this family member as a *protagonist of change* and improvement for the entire group. Specifically, the difficult child may be the one who "sees it all," and is thus holding onto (and *acting out*) the troubles in the family at large.

Discussing this concept with the entire family can be like opening a Pandora's box of dreams, fantasies, anguish, and previously unidentified memories. This is because every one of us exists inside of a context, and when we start a dialogue about our truer feelings, we risk seeing ourselves, and our relationships, in very different ways than we originally perceived them. Emotional themes that may have occurred in our parent's generation may end up surfacing, and we find ourselves running from *unresolved dilemmas* of the past.

Seen in this way, the abused child is possibly the most sensitive, and most powerful, agent of growth and change for the whole family. He or she holds the pain for everyone—pain that was unknowingly brewing beneath the surface of a seemingly healthy home. Thus, in educating ourselves, and the world, about child abuse, we are wise to search for repetitive patterns of behavior in our family. These may actually be behaviors that are motivated by fear.

Regardless of how we define it, the labeling of the abused child as the "difficult one" highlights the possibility that everyone has work to do. Simply stated, when we find that we have branded one of our family members as the "black sheep" or "dark horse," we would be wise to turn to him or her and say, "Thank you. Your behavior has me thinking about a part of my past that needs further examining."

Seen in this way, the "dark horse" may just be the "bright light" that every family needs.

How were you seen by your family members?

_____

_____

_____

_____

_____

_____

_____

_____

Did this label become a part of your adult identity? If yes, write down how or in what ways:

_____

_____

_____

_____

_____

If you could tell the members of your family of origin how you wanted to be seen in their eyes back in those days, what would you say?

_____

_____

_____

_____

_____

In the end, we come to realize that our behaviors, as negative as some of them may have been, have had an effect on other people's lives. Some of these effects have been negative. But some have had, or will have, unconscious benefits for all who are involved.

Become a Person Who Affects Others' Lives

Surviving child abuse urges us to face the paradox of the human condition. Specifically, we believe that each of us was created as unique and special, with a goal of achieving as much as possible in this life. But somewhere along the way, trauma and adversity appeared, and it brought with it the unbidden feelings of shame, guilt, self-loathing, fear, and hopelessness. Defeat became our unwelcome friend, and it filled us with sorrow. We are thus left with two choices:

1. We deny our fate. We tell ourselves we are "okay" and that everything will be alright, or

2. We reach out for help and we start on the road to recovery.

Recovery starts with education. We read books, seek out mentors and therapists, and educate ourselves about the darker parts of the world in which we were raised. In fact, the very beginning stages of therapy for survivors of abuse is known as the **education stage**. This is because, at a time when we are filled with emotional urgency and unwelcome flashbacks, we benefit from learning more about "what to expect" from our journey, and we prepare ourselves for the lessons that are yet to come. Education is less laden with emotion. It is simply data. And little by little, we collect the data in our effort to learn more about ourselves.

We learn that the forbidden dreams and fears we harbor from the past are merely uncensored reflections of what we were told about ourselves. We recount the painful parts of our story and learn that we were only children and that what happened to us was *not our fault*. It was *never* our fault. We learn that, in questioning the world through the eyes of our inner child, things we did not know then will be revealed to us when we are ready—and more emotionally able—to understand them.

And in the process of our learning, we find hope. We explore our needs and wishes with mentors, teachers, therapists, or friends who truly care. We begin to create goals for ourselves. Eventually we learn to develop a plan. This plan is our *hope in action*. We have cast ourselves into a new world filled with challenges and fears, but we are determined to find strength and power over those fears. And in the end, we find ourselves becoming a person who is now capable of affecting the lives of others.

What education have you provided for yourself?

_____

_____

_____

_____

_____

What more do you need to do in order to educate yourself further? (What are the key points still missing from your life?)

_____

_____

_____

_____

_____

How will you educate your children or other vulnerable people? What measures will you put in place and what are the key points for them to learn?

_____

_____

_____

_____

_____

Notice now how you are more emotionally and intellectually connected than you were when you first started on your road to recovery. You are in the process of healing the hurt child within. And as you heal, you are gaining the wisdom and the power to teach others. This is the cycle of giving, and it is a central part of the healing you are now experiencing.

William Blake once said,

The deeper the sorrow, the greater the joy.

One way to understand this statement is that there is redemption inside of our struggle. Sorrow strengthens our soul and forces us to become brave; it challenges us to discover the spiritual and emotional wealth that exists inside of the pain; and we educate the world on all that we are learning in the process.

Education leads to transformation. This is how sorrow works over us, reshaping our trials into triumphs. We become more open, more transparent, and more accessible to others who are in need. There is a profound connection between the lessons that life is teaching us and our ability to genuinely connect with others. The teaching is fierce. It challenges us to open our ears, our hearts, and our minds, and to drop the prejudice and fear that once blindly guided us. It asks that we finally change the narrative and the stigma that surrounds child abuse.

What has your transformation (from when you started your healing journey to now) looked like?

_____

_____

_____

_____

_____

How will you go about changing the narrative in your family, community, and culture?

_____

_____

_____

_____

_____

Each time we open a dialogue about abuse, we break the stigma and provide a voice for those who cannot speak up for themselves. The conversation is only just beginning. We must continue to tell the story, and ask the questions, until one day, the world finally hears and responds.

10

The Future

When patterns are broken, new worlds emerge.

Tuli Kupferberg

We all have an invitation buried deep within our despair. It is an invitation to restore ourselves, through courage, to a state of wholeness. Despair was our human response to pain, to loss, and to fear. Our hearts were overwhelmed, and our reality was overtaken. But now, after years of struggle to make sense of it all, we are attempting something new. We are attempting to cultivate courage. We are working toward closure. And we are discovering the unexpected grace that comes with telling our story.

The future offers us the possibility of new beginnings. But we must embrace this opportunity without self-judgment. This is because criticism constricts our soul and stifles our growth, whereas compassion expands our soul, allowing healthy love to flourish.[83] We have chosen to heal, to be survivors rather than victims. It is now time to remove some of the emotional armor that once protected us and attempt to embrace new ideas and find new ways of living.

As we journey forward, we recognize that we must reframe the concept of asking for help as an act of courage. We acknowledge the reality of our condition and we take steps to change and grow. This is our hope in action. This is our sign of strength. Far from granting victory over our abuser, we are empowering ourselves as survivors.[84]

The outcome of our healing journey depends on our ability to tolerate the discomfort that comes from facing our memories without becoming overwhelmed by them. This is not easy work, and there is no quick fix. We know that we may find ourselves, at times, regressing into childlike behaviors (our memories can seduce us back to old, familiar modes of relating.) But still we muscle forward. We know that our recovery involves restoring the healthy connection we have to our adult selves, the part of us that has the strength and the will to succeed.

The four R's to readying ourselves for the future are the following:

- Reconstructing the Story
- Reconnecting
- Revamping
- Restoring Justice

We offer a summary of each of these constructs below:

Reconstructing the Story

One important task in our journey forward is to reconstruct a new interpretation of the traumatic event(s) that happened to us. In reconstructing our story, we are making our testimony. This confession, in the presence of a loving other, brings with it new ways for us to understand and interpret the meaning of our experience. We are re-instating ourselves into the world that we lost all those years ago. The locus of control remains with us; we are in charge of our memories and we pace ourselves as needed.

EXERCISE 22

The Writing Ritual

This exercise is best completed in a safe environment with a trusted therapist or counselor.

1. Carefully, and with safe connection to a loving other, **write down** the events as you remember them. The written memory must contain three elements: the facts, your feelings, and the meaning as you understand it.
2. When you are ready, **read the story aloud**.
3. **Revise the script** with the help of your trusted counselor. During the revision process, you and your therapist can organize your recollections, until they take on a coherent structure.

4. **Begin the process of mastery**; recognize that you are no longer imprisoned by the wordlessness of the trauma. You have named the monster and now you can tame its effects.

5. **Generate possible alternative meanings** to the events that took place. This part of the exercise allows you to consider new dimensions in interpreting an old script.

Write the events as you remember them:

_____

_____

_____

_____

_____

_____

_____

_____

_____

Now revise the script with the help of a counselor or therapist:

_____

_____

_____

_____

_____

_____

_____

_____

_____

_____

_____

_____

Now generate alternative meanings:

_____

_____

_____

_____

_____

_____

_____

_____

_____

_____

When we explore the traumatic memories in the context of a safe and secure relationship, we are actually facilitating a new way for us to process and understand the event. With support, we assemble and reassemble our fragmented memories, rewriting the meaning as we go along. We see it from a different perspective, and we discover that our story is not about shame and humiliation, but about pride and dignity. We let ourselves off the hook, for as we write, we denounce what was done to us rather than own it as a shameful part of ourselves.

We are using our story as medicine. We write it down, not because we want to, but because we must.[85] Our words have become our narrative; they form a script that is deeply carved into our identity. But our story must not remain embedded there. Through careful exploration of our memories, we can begin to share with others and have the chance to rewrite parts of the story, and even imagine it having a happier ending.

Reconnection

In facing the task of creating a future, we must consider developing new relationships. The credos and myths that once guided us are no longer useful in our recovery, and it is time for us to find new and supportive attachments. We take concrete steps to deepen our alliances with those we trust, and we honor the moments when we feel safe in their company.

This is an act of great courage, and this is for two reasons:

First, we must bear the discomfort that comes from getting close to another person.

Second, we must be prepared to empathize with a friend who may be struggling with their own sorrows.

And when we do this, we find ourselves rejoining the community, transforming our fear and insecurity into care and concern for others who are hurt like us. We relate to our new friend with loving-kindness, and he relates to us likewise, as we both pass through the multitude of life's trials and joys.

Revamping

Once we have achieved a sense of safety and security, we pursue a new agenda of the things we need or want to accomplish. We either recover some of our goals and aspirations from the time before the trauma, or we discover new ambitions and set out to accomplish them.

This work is about freedom and choice—for we are no longer controlled by the voices of our past.[86] We maintain our adult presence and we entertain our ability to encounter life with greater confidence. Some of us who have survived trauma commit to teaching others how to stay safe. We become motivational speakers, writers, and teachers, for we have a story to tell. It is a story of how we moved through trauma and came out triumphant.

Looking at where you are today. What does your future look like?

_____

_____

_____

_____

What are some new goals you have as you move from trauma to triumph?

_____

_____

_____

_____

What needs to be done to achieve them?

_____

_____

_____

_____

Restoring Justice

A guiding principle in journeying forward involves the restoration of our sense of justice. This is a therapeutic approach where a meeting is organized between victim and offender in the presence of a representative of the community.[87] The aim of this coming together is for abuser and abused to share their experience of what happened; discuss the impact it had on each of them; and discern the consequences and the possible reparations to be made.

The program allows victims of abuse the chance to reclaim their voice; this time, as a survivor and not as a victim. Victims often speak of their need to re-narrate their life stories as survivors of violence. Thus, one goal of a restorative justice encounter is the change in the self-narrative.

The most frequent questions needing answers when a victim meets his or her perpetrator are:

1. Why did you do it?
2. Why did you choose me?
3. Will you attempt to do this again to me or to someone else?
4. How much remorse do you feel for the suffering that you caused me?
5. Did something similar happen to you?

Getting answers to these questions can allow a victim a chance to move forward in his or her recovery process. It affords him an active role in the judicial system; an apology and an acknowledgment of the crime; and the possibility of finding some semblance of peace, justice, and closure.

The process also ensures that an offender take responsibility for his actions, or at least attempts to understand the damage he caused to the victim(s). It aims at offering the perpetrator an opportunity to make good on the pain he caused, redeem himself, as well as prevent him from causing further harm to others.

Interventions such as these allow for a clear definition of the intense shame that was caused, and it does so in a rehabilitative and destigmatizing manner.[88] This can be part of a process of personal transformation for all people who are involved.

If you had an opportunity to meet with your offender through the restorative justice system, how would you feel, and what are some of the questions you would ask and want to know?

_____

_____

_____

_____

_____

_____

Would this allow you to find the peace you need to move forward? _____

After a meeting like this, do you think you could have compassion on yourself for everything you have been through? If the answer is no, please write down why.

_____

_____

_____

_____

Self-Compassion

Of all of the tasks that we need to accomplish in our search for a brighter future, the ability to love ourselves is by far the hardest. Hurt people hurt people; and since we have been hurt, we end up hurting ourselves. We judge and criticize, even attack, our internal sense of being, fully believing the words that we are aggressively saying beneath our breath.

But bringing compassion to our own suffering is a necessary part of our healing from abuse. It is an act of courage, as well as of generosity. It reminds us that we too are worthy and valuable. It is our guide to a healthier future, for our ability to accept love from another person is directly proportional to our capacity to love ourselves.

Self-Compassion

The following guided imagery exercise is designed to help you develop greater compassion for yourself as you journey into the future.

Try to get as comfortable as possible. Just breathe in through your nose and breathe out through your mouth fully and completely. As you breathe in, imagine yourself on a long road with nothing but trees lining the path.

Suddenly, you see a young child, sitting alone, by the side of this long, empty road. They are lost and do not know how to find their way home. In this moment, you sense the sorrow and the fear in their heart.

Now is the time to radiate loving-kindness to the child in front of you.

Continue to breathe in naturally...and completely. Recognize the compassion that is in your heart and extend it to them...

When you feel ready, let this image fade and allow yourself to see the child you used to be take his place on that road. You know their suffering; you know what they have been through. You know how lost they feel. Offer them the same loving-kindness you offered the child who came before them.

How does it feel to give that inner child your love?

_____

_____

_____

_____

_____

_____

This is the beginning of learning self-compassion. Notice that it may come at a cost to your sense of comfort. Psychologist and professor Kristin Neff calls this a **back draft**. It refers to the pain that arises when we give ourselves kindness and compassion. The term originates from firefighters to describe the paradoxically devastating effect that fire has when all of the available oxygen has been used up, and new oxygen has been introduced through an open door or window. When we start using self-compassion, a new door opens in our heart and the old pain and fear rush out. Do not fear the back draft, it is actually a paradoxical sign that we are getting better.

Tears can come through utilizing some of these meditative techniques. Anger, fear, and re-traumatization are at the core of our tears.

Ask yourself, "What do I need right now to move forward in a safe way as I do this necessary healing work?"

_____

_____

_____

_____

_____

_____

Tell yourself that this is just a back draft of old emotional residue that is finding its way out through the opened door in your heart.

- Pay attention to the way your body is reacting, and give that part of your body a supportive touch or virtual hug.
- Remind yourself that you have been through this before and that this moment shall pass.
- Tell yourself: "I am worthy. I am deserving of love. And I am not alone."

What future work do you think you need to do to find compassion for the child inside of you?

_____

_____

_____

_____

_____

_____

Everybody responds to traumatic memories differently. Allow yourself to have whatever experience you had, and offer yourself kindness. You are on your way to achieving a form of closure.

Closure

The term **closure** derives from a branch of psychology known as Gestalt therapy.[89] It denotes our need for clear and concise answers to the ambiguous information that our brain receives throughout the lifespan. Our brain does not like uncertainty; it is always attempting to *close the gaps* in the things it perceives.[90] It wants to "make meaning" out of confusing moments. We thus impose a narrative on the incoming information that we receive. Sometimes our narrative can lead to negative assumptions, but it does create a sense of relief for the confused mind.

The term is now utilized by other schools of psychological thought. Specifically, in the field of trauma and bereavement, closure represents our human need to make sense of the negative experiences we endured and ultimately transform them into actions that will help us move forward. It is an act or a wish for the completion, or resolution, of a difficult time in life.

Understood in this way, our search for closure can help us with the complex, painful, and confusing emotions that arise from our traumatic memories. We are seeking understanding, peace, and a sense of finality. We want that part of our lives to be over. It is indeed a bold aspiration, but we are determined to place this part of our story somewhere where it no longer defines or overwhelms us.

We offer here the following steps for you to consider as you start on *your* path to achieving closure:

- Connect with others who understand your pain or sorrow (therapists and support groups).
- Learn to embrace these feelings for as long as you need.
- Open a new door or window in your heart to let these feelings and fears finally escape.
- Support those who hurt in similar ways as you.
- Educate the world so this will never happen again.

───────────── EXERCISE 24 ─────────────

The Letter

Healing is a restorative process that invokes wisdom through ritual, and rituals have been our most powerful tool of survival throughout these very difficult years. Through ritual we attune ourselves to our culture, our traditions, and our community; but we also attune with our inner world—the world our soul inhabits.[91] Rituals offer us a place of containment. Like sacred alchemy, rituals create a holding space for us to refine and purify our sense of self. In this holding space we allow our anguish out. Nothing is held back.

To complete this ritual, we ask you to write a letter to your abuser, or to your trauma. You can be as honest and as vulnerable as you wish—no one will see what you have written. Use the empty page as a canvas on which to write your truth, as well as the wisdom you acquired on your healing journey.

Write your letter on a separate piece of paper.

When you have finished, do what you must with the letter. Burn it, bury it, place it in a safe for your future self to read. But release it from the bondage of shame and fear that once inhabited your inner psyche. You are healing; and the shame, fear, and anguish no longer belong inside of you.

What does closure look or feel like to you?

_____

_____

_____

_____

_____

_____

In an ideal world, what does your future look like and what do you still need to do in order to achieve this important goal?

_____

_____

_____

_____

_____

Pain bears its own cure, like that of a child.

Jelaluddin Rumi

We learn from the prophetic words of the Sufi poet Rumi that pain cleanses our heart as it challenges our mind. Our questioning never ceases, but through our questions, self-expansion and dominion over our sadness and trauma can and do prevail.

How we deal with our trauma is relative, and it will define its impact on our future. We can bury it deep within the psyche and pretend it never happened, or we can bravely face it. After reading this book and working through the exercises, we hope that we, as survivors, can learn to sit beneath pain's unwelcome shadow until we learn what it came here to teach. Many of us were told, time and again, to "get over it," to "move on," or to "forget." Sadly, these common directives only create greater suffering. This is because our charge, as survivors of trauma, is to acknowledge that what happened to us is now a part of us. It is embedded in our DNA.

Thus, we wrestle with our demons and we wrestle with our angels. And through the long night of struggle, we discover ways to integrate the effects of our trauma into a new and healthier sense of self. We learn to *embrace the pain* so that we can eventually *place the pain* somewhere where it no longer hurts us in ways it once did.

We now have the tools of self-compassion and psychological understanding and, with these tools, we know we will never fall again. This is the future.

This is the beginning of our new life.

Final Word

You have worked your way through the exercises and essays in this book. Congratulations to you. There may have been times when you felt like you were walking in unwelcome territory. Memories and emotions that were buried long ago were likely reactivated, causing you to feel unsettled and afraid.

From a biological perspective, some of the material you read may have created temporary changes in sleep or appetite, agitation, or poor focus, as well the resurgence of unwelcome memories. This is normal; it is the body's response to trauma, and sometimes we feel worse before we feel better.

You may wish to seek out your own psychotherapy as you now enter into a new stage of recovery. A good therapist, a true healer, can help you to remain steadfast as you wrestle the unwelcome reminders of your past. He or she can prop you up and help you to see the infinite possibilities that exist inside of you.

Having reached the end of this workbook, we pray that the light of a new day will eventually come. And when that day arrives, you may place the unwelcome remnants of your old life down, for they serve no purpose in this new land. Your arrival here comes from the choice you made to finally heal the wounds of the past.

Welcome. May elevation of soul and healing of body be yours in the new life you have chosen to live.

Endnotes

1. Bessel Van Der Kolk, *The Body Keeps the Score; Brain, Mind and Body in the Healing of Trauma*, New York: Penguin Books, 2014.

2. Richard Rohr, *Falling Upward: A Spirituality for the Two Halves of Life*, San Francisco, CA: Jossey-Bass, 2011.

3. Patrick Carnes, *Out of the Shadows: Understanding Sexual Addiction*, Center City, MT: Hazelden Publishing, 2001.

4. Joseph Soloveitchik, *Out of the Whirlwind: Essays on Mourning, Suffering and the Human Condition*, Brooklyn, NY: KTAV Publishing House, Inc., 2003.

5. Jolande Jacobi, *The Psychology of Carl Jung*, New Haven, CT: Yale University Press, 1973.

6. A. W. Bendig, "Factor Analytic Scales of Covert and Overt Hostility," *Journal of Consulting Psychology* 26, no. 2 (1962): 200.

7. Maggie Scarf, *Intimate Partners: Patterns in Love and Marriage*, New York: Ballantine Books, 1987.

8. Matthew McKay, Jeffrey Brantley, and Jeffrey Wood, *The Dialectical Behavior Therapy Workbook: Practical DBT Exercises for Learning Mindfulness, Interpersonal Effectiveness, and Distress Tolerance*, Oakland, CA: New Harbinger Publications, Inc., 2019.

9. John Illman, *Use Your Brain to Beat Depression: The Complete Guide to Understanding and Tackling Depressive Illness*, London, UK: Cassell & Co., 2004.

10. Judith Herman, *Trauma and Recovery: The Aftermath of Violence—From Domestic Abuse to Political Power*, New York: Basic Books, 1992.

11. Van Der Kolk, *The Body Keeps the Score*.

12. J. D. Bremner and M. Narayan, "The Effects of Stress on Memory and The Hippocampus Throughout the Life Cycle: Implications for Childhood Development and Aging," *Developmental Psychopathology* 10 (1998): 871–886.

13. McKay, *The Dialectical Behavior Therapy Workbook*.

14. Beverly James, *Handbook for Treatment of Attachment-Trauma Problems in Children*, New York: The Free Press, 1994.

15. Norman Fried, *Reclaiming Humanity: A Guide to Maintaining the Inner World of the Child Facing Ongoing Trauma*, Brooklyn, NY: Urim Publications, 2017.

16. Norman Murray, R. Koby, and Bessel van Der Kolk, "The Effects of Abuse on Children's Thoughts," Chapter 4 in *Psychological Trauma*, Washington D.C.: American Psychiatric Press, 1987.

17. J. Ostroff, et al., *Hope and Uncertainty: Family Responses to Completing Childhood Cancer Treatment*, Proceedings of the Annual Meeting of the APA: New York, 1995.

18. H. Selye, "Stress and the General Adaptation Syndrome," *British Medical Journal* 1 (1950): 1383–92.

19. Terry Philpot, *Understanding Child Abuse: The Partners of Child sex Offenders Tell Their Stories*, London, UK: Routledge, 2009.

20. Nathan Spiteri, *Toy Cars,* Three Australia: Little Birds Press, 2021.

21. Charles Simpkinson, and Anne Simpkinson, *Sacred Stories: A Celebration of the Power of Stories to Transform and Heal*, San Francisco, CA: Harper San Francisco, 1993.

22. Philpot, *Understanding Child Abuse.*

23. Fried, *Reclaiming Humanity.*

24. James, *Handbook for Treatment of Attachment-Trauma Problems in Children.*

25. Scarf, *Intimate Partners.*

26. John Gottman, *Why Marriages Succeed or Fail: And How You Can Make Yours Last*, New York: Simon & Schuster, 1995.

27. Pauline Rose Clance, *The Imposter Phenomenon: When Success Makes You Feel Like a Fake*, Atlanta, GA: Peachtree Press, 1985.

28. Judith S. Beck, *Cognitive Therapy: Basics and Beyond*, New York: Guilford Press, 1995.

29. Paul Gilbert, "The Evolved Basis and Adaptive Functions of Cognitive Distortions," *British Journal of Medical Psychology* 71, no, 9 (1998): 447–63.

30. Scarf, *Intimate Partners.*

31. Philpot, *Understanding Child Abuse.*

32. Maggie Scarf, *Intimate Worlds: Life Inside the Family*, New York: Random House, 1995.

33. Michael Pollan, *How to Change Your Mind: What the New Science of Psychedelics Teaches Us About Consciousness, Depression, and Transcendence*, New York: Penguin, 2018.

34. Herman, *Trauma and Recovery.*

35. Robert B. Cialdini, and Melanie R. Trost, "Social Influence: Social Norms, Conformity, and Compliance," In *The Handbook of Social Psychology*, New York: McGrawHill, 1998.

36. John Bowlby, *Attachment and Loss*, New York: Basic Books, 1969.

37. Scarf, *Intimate Partners.*

38. Beverly Engel, *It Wasn't Your Fault: Freeing Yourself from the Shame of Childhood Abuse with the Power of Self-Compassion*, New York: New Harbinger Publications, 2015.

39. Van Der Kolk, *The Body Keeps the Score.*

40. Richard Lane, Claudia Subic-Wrana, Leslie Greenberg, and Iftah Yovel, "The Role of Enhanced Emotional Awareness in Promoting Changes Across Psychotherapy Modalities," *Journal of Psychotherapy Integration* 32, no. 2 (2022): 131–150.

41. Marsha Linehan, *DBT Skills Training Manual* (2nd ed,) New York: Guilford Press, 2015.

42. Sigmund Freud, *The Ego and the Id: The Standard Edition*, New York: WW Norton, 1923.

43. James, *Handbook for Treatment of Attachment-Trauma Problems in Children.*

44. Robert Greene, *The 48 Paws of Power*, New York: Viking, 1998.

45. *The Soncino Talmud; The Book of Oral Jewish Law*, London, UK: The Sorincino Press, 1948.

46. Fried, *Reclaiming Humanity.*

47. Friends in Recovery, *The 12 Steps—A Way Out: A Spiritual Process for Healing*, Scotts Valley, AZ: RPI Publishing, 2012.

48. Spiteri, *Toy Cars.*

49. Freud, *The Ego and the Id.*

50. Beck, *Cognitive Therapy.*

51. Patrick Carnes, *Out of The Shadows: Understanding Sexual Addiction*, Center City, MT: Hazelden Publishing, 2001.

52. Spiteri, *Toy Cars.*

53. Lenore Terr, *Unchained Memories: True Stories of Traumatic Memories, Lost and Found*, New York: Basic Books, 1994.

54. Mark Epstein, *Thoughts Without a Thinker: Psychotherapy from a Buddhist Perspective*, New York: Basic Books, 1995.

55. Mary Frances O'Connor, *The Grieving Brain: The Surprising Science of how We Learn from Love and Loss*, New York: Harper Collins, 2022.

56. Carl G. Jung, *Memories, Dreams, Reflections*, New York Random House, 1963.

57. Norman Freid, *The Angel Letters: Lessons that Dying Can Teach Us About Living*, Chicago, IL: Rowman & Littlefield, 2007.

58. Scarf, *Intimate Partners.*

59. Francis Weller, *The Wild Edge of Sorrow: Rituals of Renewal and The Sacred Work of Grief*, Berkeley, CA: North Atlantic Books, 2015.

60. Clarissa Pinkola-Estes, *Women Who Run with the Wolves: Myths and Stories of the Wild Woman Archetype*, New York: Ballantine Books, 1995.

61. Ellen Bass, and Laura Davis, *The Courage to Heal: A Guide for Women Survivors of Child Sexual Abuse*, New York: Harper & Row Publishers, 1994.

62. Shakti Gawain, *Return to the Garden: A Journey of Discovery*, New Delhi, India: Nataraj Publishing, 1989.

63. David Sheff, *Clean: Overcoming Addiction and Ending America's Greatest Tragedy*, Boston, MA: Houghton Mufflin Harcourt, 2013.

64. Ronald Ruden, *The Craving Brain: A Bold New Approach to Breaking Free from Drug-Addiction, Overeating, Alcoholism and Gambling*, New York: Harper Perennial, 2000.

65. Patrick Carnes, *Out of The Shadows: Understanding Sexual Addiction*, Center City, MT: Hazelden Publishing, 2001.

66. Carlo DiClementi, *Addiction and Change: How Addictions Develop and Addicted People Recover*, New York: The Guilford Press, 2003.

67. Addiction Center, "Subsidiary of Recovery World LLC," AddictionCenter.com.

68. Judith Grisel, *Never Enough: The Neuroscience and Experience of Addiction.* New York: Doubleday Books, 2019.

69. "Obesity and Overweight," World Health Organization, June 9, 2021.

70. Ronald David Laing, *The Divided Self*, Middlesex, England: Penguin Books, 1971.

71. Friends in Recovery, *The 12 Steps—A Way Out.*

72. Patrick Carnes, *Out of the Shadows: Understanding Sexual Addiction*, Center City, MT: Hazelden Publishing, 2001.

73. John W. Crandall, "Pathological Nurturance: The Root of Marital Discord," *Journal of Family Counseling* 4 (1976): 62–68.

74. Van Der Kolk, *The Body Keeps the Score.*

75. Fried, *Reclaiming Humanity*.

76. Bremner, "The Effects of Stress on Memory and the Hippocampus Throughout the Life Cycle: Implications for Childhood Development and Aging."

77. Herman, *Trauma and Recovery*.

78. Van Der Kolk, *The Body Keeps the Score*.

79. A. Gangemi, M. Daho, and F. Mancini, "Emotional Reasoning and Psychopathology," *Brain Science* 11, no. 4 (2021): 471.

80. Antonis Hatzigeorgiadis and Evangelos Galanis, "Self-Talk Effectiveness and Attention," *Journal of Current Opinion in Psychology* 16 (2017): 138–142.

81. Philpot, *Understanding Child Abuse*.

82. Philpot, *Understanding Child Abuse*.

83. Viktor Frankl, *Man's Search for Meaning*, New York: Beacon Press, 2000.

84. Weller, *The Wild Edge of Sorrow*.

85. Simpkinson, *Sacred Stories*.

86. Irvin D. Yalom, *Existential Psychotherapy*, New York: Basic Books, 1980.

87. Daniel W. Van Ness, Karen Heetderks-Strong, Jonathan Derby, and Lynette Parker, *Restore Justice: An Introduction to Restorative Justice*, London, UK: Routledge, 2014.

88. Alex Lloyd and Jo Borill, "Examining the Effectiveness of Restorative Justice in Reducing Victims' Post-Traumatic Stress," *Psychological Inquiry and Law* 13 (2019): 77–89.

89. Rosalba Raffagnino, "Gestalt Therapy Effectiveness: A Systematic Review of Empirical Evidence," *Open Journal of Social Sciences* 7, no. 6 (2019).

90. Pollan, *How to Change Your Mind*.

91. Carl G. Jung, *Modern Man in Search of a Soul*, New York: Harcourt, Brace & World, Inc., 1933.

About the Authors

After receiving his PhD in clinical and pediatric psychology from Emory University, **Dr. Norman J. Fried** served as the chief psychologist for the Children's Cancer Centers and the Division of Pediatric Hematology/Oncology at Northwell Health and Winthrop University Hospitals for 20 years. His academic appointments include assistant professor in pediatrics and psychiatry at New York University Medical School, adjunct assistant professor of pastoral counseling at the Jewish Theological Seminary/Columbia University, and fellow in clinical and pediatric psychology at Harvard Medical School.

Now in full-time private practice as a grief and trauma specialist, Norman lectures on the practice of psychotherapy with critically and terminally ill children and their families at conferences across the US and Europe. Additionally, he is a disaster mental health specialist for the American Red Cross of greater New York. He is the author of four books, including *The Childhood Trauma Recovery Workbook for Adults*. Additionally, he is a regular contributor on crisis intervention and recovery for television and news shows, including *Dr. Phil*, Fox News, BBC World News, NBC News, and the Bravo channel.

Nathan Spiteri is a filmmaker, actor, and writer. He is also a sexual abuse survivor, TEDx speaker, activist, and advocate. Through intensive therapy and group work, Nathan now educates people on the stigma of child sexual abuse and its relation to addiction and substance abuse, and helps other survivors find closure and move forward with their lives while raising awareness of men's mental health.

Nathan works with a number of charitable organizations both in the US and Australia. He is currently the global ambassador for the Child Liberation Foundation, a foundation with the goal to eliminate child sex trafficking around the world. He also works with the Aussies Say No More Campaign as part of the global No More Campaign, Menslink, and Survivors and Mates Support Network, one of Australia's leading associations for male survivors of child sexual abuse. His memoir, *Toy Cars*, is a powerful account of survival and inspiration.